A Book Series

Perfect At Last
WEIGHT

Evolutionary Perspective's Guide on
Fasting for Optimum Weight & Healing

SECOND EDITION

by Josephine Grace Rojo Tan, MD

Table of Contents

Copyright 1

Dedication 3

Acknowledgement 5

About The Author 7

Disclaimer 10

INTRODUCTION 13

Truths About Eating and Fasting 19

Fat-Storing Versus Fat- Losing Mechanism 27

Why Meal Timing Matters 40

The Basics of Fasting 45

Dry Fasting, Wet Fasting & Fluids 50

Who Can Fast 67

Who Cannot Fast 71

Extended Fasting 77

Intermittent Fasting 87

Factors Affecting Fat Loss While Fasting 92

Foods that Enhance Fat Loss 108

   Approved Green List of Foods You Can Eat Freely 111

Foods to Avoid in Fat Loss 115

   Unapproved Red List Foods to be Avoided 119

No Cheating, Make Plans Instead 123

What About Exercise	127
Weight Loss Plateau	131
Why & How I Started Fasting	137
Fasting Thoughts and Tips	145
Other Benefits of Fasting	152
Summary and Pearls	156
Frequently Asked Questions	162
REFERENCES/SUGGESTED READINGS:	169
Different 20-gram carbohydrates	173
Basal Metabolic Index Chart	176
Sample Intermittent Fasting Schedules	178
Sample Short-term EF Schedules	180
#JGCRojoFoodList	181
Let's Start This Journey Together	183
List and Recipe of Easy, Affordable	189
Low Carbohydrate Dessert	191
Low Carb Cooking and Baking	192
DCR Protocol	193
Author's Notes	199

Copyright

Copyright © 2023 by Josephine Grace Rojo Tan

All rights reserved. This book or any portion thereof may not be reproduced or used in any manner whatsoever without the written permission of the publisher and author except for the use of brief quotations in a book review or scholarly journal.

First Printing: 2023

www.jgrtanmd.com

Dedication

To my first family, *Papa, Maming, Aunt Angelie & Uncle Jerome*, brothers *Alvin, Andrew & Bappy*, and my beloved sister *Cath*, thank you.

And to my chosen family, my husband, *Kenneth Bryan*, I cannot thank God enough for you, and this book is one of my attempts in expressing that gratitude.

Acknowledgement

Special thanks to the admins and moderators of our Facebook pages Life Without Rice and Low Carb Feasting and Fasting Community for the patience, learnings, and kindness to help our online community sustain our LCF way of life.

About The Author

My name is *Grace,* and I am a practicing medical doctor by profession. I took Bachelor of Arts in Psychology in college before I proceeded to medicine. The second I learned about how we evolved as humans, was the moment I developed both curiosity and fascination with how our body continuously responds like cavemen even to modern-day challenges. Say for example, a traffic situation leaving one unable to do anything but be still. Such scenario triggers anxiety and sends modern men to resort to their *fight or flight response.* Thus, blood instinctively flows to the hands and legs, in preparation to either engage in a physical fight or to run for one's life *(like how homo sapiens did millions of years ago),* making the legs restless for not being able to do anything, other than sit still and endure the traffic-induced pain. And as I went on, I realized that this holds true in many aspects of our day-to-day living, especially with our eating pattern.

We are in the 21st century but our body still functions the way it used to for the last thousands if not millions of years of its genetic existence. Like many of you, I had issues with my weight for as long as I can remember. I have tried so many diet regimes but with no sustainable results. Growing up, I have always been on the heavier side. I am 5-foot, 5 inches tall and the heaviest I have recorded weighing was 141 pounds.

Quite certainly, I have weighed more, but I just didn't have the courage to weigh myself during those times. I always look back to a transient time in high school and college where I considered to have been at my slimmest weight of 121 pounds. This may sound like it isn't a struggle since I never really reached the obese scale, but the truth is, there is a real challenge in trying to lose weight when you are already within what is considered as "*normal*", albeit non-ideal self.

My relationship with food is just something that I could not get a hold of. And it has deep roots since the same is a struggle with the rest of my family. Food has always been a source of comfort, happiness, and it is a part of every celebration. Skipping a meal is just out of the deal. Unintentional skipped meals are compensated immediately right after. But tragedy occurred in our family. The loss of my father and three of his other siblings in their early 50s consecutively for four years due to lifestyle disease, had me question my unhealthy habits and seriously thought about improving my overall wellness, starting with my weight.

And as I go back and see it from an *evolutionary perspective,* backed up by scientific evidence from my study of medicine, what I needed to do became clear. I did what nobody in my world thought I could ever do. And in a month's time, I achieved the body weight that I thought would only be in my dreams. From 140+ pounds, I became 115-118 and a BMI of 19-19.5 and eventually stabilized to the mid BMI of 20-21 with more lean body mass and lower visceral fat mass. I always have the energy and the endurance to do my work as a surgeon, among many other things, without difficulty than I used to have because of excess fats and low muscle mass.

With determination, adequate knowledge, and proper mindset, your body weight can be perfect at last too.

Disclaimer

The information written in this book is from the best of the author's knowledge at the time of production with the sincerest intention to help. This book only intends to serve as a guide and does not intend to replace the specific medical advice given to each patient by his or her own physician. It will not substitute the medications currently prescribed to the reader for a specific illness.

Any dietary and lifestyle recommendations mentioned in this book are the personal view of the author. Readers are strongly advised to conduct their own research and consultations to verify the applicability of the texts written in this guide to each personal case. The author does not and will not derive any financial gain from organizations or companies mentioned in these texts. As of this writing, and as far as the knowledge of the author is concerned, there has been no medical emergency associated with the recommendations in this book.

The reader is solely responsible for any lifestyle changes he or she may wish to proceed with after reading this book. It is strongly recommended that consultation with your trusted physician should be done first prior to embarking on any lifestyle change, especially for people with existing medical illness.

No copyright infringement is intended on the photos used in this book. Credits are given to the owners and sites where the photos were taken.

Should there be any inadvertent copyright infringement committed, kindly contact the author so immediate rectification may be undertaken.

INTRODUCTION

Understanding Where We Came From

At least 700 million years ago, the closest ancestor of humans roamed the earth. They feed on whatever fresh fruits and vegetables available on their given location at that specific season. You see, once all produce is consumed in that area, it might take some time before they can eat again.

There will be days and even weeks of starvation and yet, they didn't die of hunger, they continued to live and persisted.

Fast-forward to 800,000 years ago, our more developed ancestors learned about controlled fire and eventually evolved to discover cooking. It allowed them to consume and derive more nutrients from the previously uncooked and raw food sources which made them stronger, wiser, and better. As hunters and gatherers, they can already eat meat and cook some variety of crops in addition to their previous diet. This led to a more advanced brain functioning.

But despite this, still, there was no mode of food preservation then and whatever they got from days of hunting, must be eaten in a short period of time to avoid spoilage. And what will follow are again prolonged days of hunger and even no food at all, but they continued to live, until the next hunt is successful, and everyone is once again fed.

Thus, if you try to imagine their normal day, breakfast isn't part of the usual deal, and dinner comes early since the danger of the night forces them to seek for a safe shelter away from predators, making their daily *window period of eating* very limited and far from our current time frame of eating, that is, eating whenever we are awake.

It's only about 10,000 BC that the transition from *hunter-gatherer stage* shifted to *stationary farming*. By this time, humans no longer need to travel places and hunt long distances just to eat. Instead, they can eat whenever crops and livestock are already set for harvest, signifying periods of abundance. In between, there are still intermittent periods of scarcity wherein *fasting*, just like hundreds of thousands of years ago, were considered a normal part of day-to-day lives. As our ancestors, they too are physically fit, active, and muscular. No evidence showing signs of obesity or problems associated therewith like diabetes, hypertension, or tumors. Causes of death are mostly related to old age, trauma in nature, accidents, or infection. This timeline comprised more than 99% of human evolution that eventually shaped our genetic makeup. The genetic changes that were incorporated during those times practically explains why our body responds instinctively the way it does, and expectedly, adapted to *fasting* as it already became a normal part of life.

By the 18th century, approximately just about 200 years ago, (which is a *very small part* in the overall human evolution), *advanced farming* began and a widespread availability of wheat, maize, potatoes, and rice as house staples became a norm.

With various food preservation techniques, people can now basically eat at any time they want. Food is available 24 hours a day, seven days a week, all year round. And what has become of our body that was used to scarcity and not of abundance? Did it evolve fast enough to adapt to these changes in our lifestyle brought about by industrialization? Can the human body accommodate all the modern-day food innovations that aim to prevent us all from ever experiencing hunger? Unfortunately, it did not.

To illustrate this impact further, it is said that if we are to compress our evolutionary history as humans to ONE YEAR (*of eating mostly meat, occasional root crops, fruits, and vegetables, with lots of fasting in between*), we've only started eating rice, wheat and grains YESTERDAY and just began consuming table sugar and fructose syrups AN HOUR ago. No wonder our body appears to be in shock if we eat the way that the majority of the population eat nowadays.

Our body was stuck in an era designed for fasting. Our culinary expertise and kitchen expanded too fast for our genes to adapt.

Thus, what do you think will happen to all the modern-day food that our anciently wired body consumes? It doesn't know what to do with all that but store it the only way it knows how - as lots and lots of body fats. Our body kept on storing **fats** (just like it used to *in preparation for the inevitable days of scarcity* that was the norm for thousands of years). It stores foods in the form of fats every chance it gets in time for the supposedly *regularly occurring* periods of *fasting*, that, as we know now, will most likely never happen.

This food abundance is now a plague causing illnesses in various forms that usually starts with one beginning to lean towards the *"healthier and chubbier"* side, then becomes a little overweight and before you know it, nothing fits anymore. And suddenly, you are already in Obese Class II. From then on, it can spiral down to co-morbidities associated with obesity like diabetes, hypertension, tumors, chronic back pain, arthritis, asthma, heart attack, kidney failure, stroke, and many more.

You see, modern-day humans are born and raised with a mindset of avoiding hunger at all costs, by parents who were also born and raised by those who define a minimum daily living decent when able to eat at least three times a day. To eat even if you are not hungry simply because it is already time to eat. And what is the result? Millions are now suffering from lifestyle diseases brought about by too much and too frequent eating habits that are far from how our body used to operate.

If only we can go back to the way we were, maybe we can have the best of the current world, with enough safety net for accidents, antibiotics for dreaded infections, and a physique that can withstand all the diseases brought about by improper food intake. It may sound counterintuitive, but in an era where everyone is maximizing the availability of food, we must also make a conscious effort to limit our intake especially when we still have stored fats to lose. And by finishing this book, I hope that in a way or two, we can make it come true.

CHAPTER I

Truths About Eating and Fasting
What we need to accept as humans

"Health and healing will follow fasting."

-Jentezen Franklin

Yes, the foundation of the evolutionary perspective's view in attaining our ideal weight is by incorporating fasting in our way of life.

For other people who have what we call the "skinny genes", the ones who frequent the buffet table but do not seem to ever gain a pound, getting fat is a far-out problem, thus fasting simply for weight loss is not for them. This is because they belong to the 50% of the population whose genes evolved and adapted to the modern-day food intake. Mind you, despite thinking that those 50% are the "lucky ones", it is also not without a catch. As what you will understand later in this series, the impact of too much food intake for those that don't get fat can be hidden until it is too late. And so, for those who have trouble attaining and maintaining a normal weight, one must accept that fasting is a natural phenomenon throughout human existence that we must also embark on.

Living in this modern world where food comes in abundance, *fasting* is a taboo. Many people just cannot comprehend how one would ever consider engaging in it. People have different and often negative views and beliefs about *eating and fasting* that, when asked further, have very little scientific explanation as back up.

The following are the **uncommon truths** about fasting and common attitude towards food that a lot of us can benefit from knowing.

Fasting will not kill you, eating all the time will.

If you think about it, metabolic diseases such as diabetes, heart disease, stroke, and to some extent, cancers, which are all related to lifestyle and eating, cause more deaths than any other disease globally, as published in the latest data by World Health Organization (WHO).

Although fasting is not synonymous to starvation, note that even the latter doesn't even score among the significant causes of death. If one eats 3x a day, 365 days a year, that is already 1,095 meals a year. Say you fast for a day, thus making it 1,092, do you really think it will make such a negative difference in your health?

It is quite amusing that those who haven't fasted are those who are certain that it cannot be done. Not because they have tried it, but simply because they are not open to it.

If you come to think of it, *fasting* is being practiced by millions worldwide. It is even a part of most religious, health, and philosophical disciplines. Fasting is even advocated as part of natural healing during the times of Hippocrates, the father of medicine. If fasting kills, do you think humanity would survive this long?

Fasting will not lead to muscle wasting.

Contrary to the common misconception, fasting will not lead to muscle wasting. During our days as cavemen, our muscles are essential in our quest for food. Thus, our body adapted greatly in such a way that our muscles will not be compromised during the time that we are still looking for food and need it the most. Instead, our body has other energy sources stored specifically reserved for times like fasting. Thus, you can be sure your muscles will be well preserved.

Breakfast is NOT the most important meal.

You might have heard and believed the opposite of this statement, but I hope you know that line was made popular by a company selling cereals made specifically to make breakfast convenient, with the goal of profit and not your health.

Breakfast, as we know now, is the meal we eat in the morning, usually before 10:00 AM. And it is okay to eat it. But it is important for you to recognize why you are eating it. Is it because you haven't eaten the night before? Or you have no other time to eat the rest of the day? Or that you will engage in an energy-requiring task that your current stores of fats cannot take? Or is it because you are just used to eating breakfast without really thinking about why?

At this point, I want you to see that eating simply because it is time to eat is NOT ideal and is very risky for your health. And the most important meal could be any meal if you eat it when your body (*and soul*) really needs it the most.

And yes, breakfast, if you must consider it as the most important, shouldn't be limited to mornings. The first meal you eat when you break your fast, whenever that may be, can in fact, can be called *breakfast*.

Small frequent meals will NOT lead to fat loss

When eating, it is not just the actual calories that make you gain weight. Whenever you eat, your pancreas secretes insulin and turns on the fat-storing mechanism switch in your body. Thus, eating small frequent meals will not lead to weight loss simply because you will have *persistent high insulin* level in your blood, putting you in a state of perpetual fat-storing mode and never in a fat-burning state.

Any amount of weight loss some experiences are due to water loss and are usually just temporary.

Low-fat, low-calorie diet lowers metabolism.

Metabolism is unique for everyone. It is a function of both body composition and activity. Unfortunately, eating a low-calorie, low-fat diet for a long time won't boost your metabolism, instead it will only make it slower. Prolonged intake of such low-calorie diet will have detrimental effects both on your metabolism and overall well-being, as what happened in the subjects in a starvation experiment done among males who were fed on low-calorie, and mostly carbohydrate, diet.

The symptoms of "hypoglycemia" when skipping meals are mostly caused by other factors other than low blood sugar.

One of the common fears of people on fasting is the risk of having a hypoglycemic episode or critically low level of blood sugar. While a low normal blood sugar is good especially once you are already adapted to fasting and are relying on a fuel source other than sugar (*yes, you can still live normally even if your sugar is low because it is not the only kind of fuel your body can use to function*), the commonly feared symptoms consisting of dizziness, tremors, and weakness are not actually due to hypoglycemia. These are mainly due to dehydration and/or electrolyte imbalance and can easily be addressed by intake of table salt and water. Dangerous hypoglycemia is seen among those who fast, eating low carb, and taking anti-hyperglycemic medications without proper guidance.

Fasting for less than 24 hours rarely causes worrisome results.

When doing an extended fast, electrolytes-rich supplements are mostly recommended for those who will continue to engage in normal physical daily activity. Doing so will make fasting adaptation a breeze. Specifics will be discussed in the succeeding chapters.

Fasting doesn't make you malnourished, overeating will.

Malnourishment refers to both being underweight and overweight. As fasting leads to weight loss, there is little evidence that it can lead to *undernourishment* simply because it is a voluntary process. Thus, when one already attains their goal weight, they can simply break their fast; establish a normal eating habit in such a way that they maintain their ideal weight. On the other hand, overeating as evidenced by steadily increasing number of lifestyle diseases, simply signifies improper and unhealthy kind of nourishment and yes, that is still under the definition of *malnourishment*.

Fasting is healthy when done right.

Weight loss may be the most noticeable effect of fasting, but it is not the only benefit you can get. Research shows that fasting can lead to longevity, can reverse diabetes and hypertension, decrease tumor growth, heal diseases related to inflammation and even lessen the risk of developing cancer, among many others.

For one to know the details on how to fast safely and effectively, is the goal of this book.

CHAPTER 2

Fat-Storing Versus Fat- Losing Mechanism
Understanding how fats are made and burned

"The best of all medicines is resting and fasting."

-Benjamin Franklin

As plain as it may sound, for those with genetic predisposition on fat buildup, (*the estimated 50% we've talked about in the first part*), consuming more than what the body needs will lead to weight gain in the form of fats. Each person has his own **Basal Metabolic Rate** (BMR), also known as the required resting energy expenditure. This is the number of calories your body is burning even if you are not doing anything. These calories will be needed by your thinking brain, pumping heart, working liver, digesting intestines, breathing lungs, warmth in your skin, and all the other parts of your body that are involuntarily working, even while you are sleeping. At an average, BMR is about 25 kcal/kg of body weight. Your BMR will dictate the minimum caloric requirement you need even when you are doing nothing. Any additional physical or mental work or any form of stress will need additional energy, thereby increasing your caloric requirement.

Say for example, a 35-year-old woman within normal BMI, weighing 55 kg and standing 5'5" with a very sedentary lifestyle, will have a BMR of 1,555 kcal. If she continues to consume more than her daily BMR, plus the 10% necessary for digestion, those excess foods will pile up and become body fats or in the form of tumors or masses.

Since it is not a common practice to calculate food intake on a day-to-day basis, often, we eat more than the amount we need. Unknowingly, the lady in our example, if she belongs to the population of *fat builders*, can slide from normal to overweight without noticing when it happened.

If you were able to perfectly balance your food intake, BMR, and physical activity since you were young, and do not have any metabolic problems, most likely you are at your most ideal body weight and are no longer in need of this book for weight-management purposes.

However, if you are like many of us who have been piling up fats in all places while living this beautiful life, you will realize that even if you try to eat less, the fats just don't easily go away. There may be times you feel that after a few days of "*dieting*" you lose weight. But the moment you go back to your normal eating habits, all the weight just comes back in. Thus as a result, you stop what you do, continue to eat, and be frustrated with how your body is transforming. It is because the initial weight loss is not true fat loss but just water loss.

Because you see, the moment that you have stored fats, those fats become the least accessible form of energy that cannot be easily burned with simple reduction in food intake.

It is during this time that you must consider reducing not the amount of food that you eat, but more importantly, reducing the frequency of your meals and/or choosing what kind of food to eat. We must understand that no matter how much we are used to eating all the time, it is simply NOT how nature intends our body to function, thus the weight gain we hate so badly becomes inevitable.

In addition, we must understand that as impossible as it may seem, the less calories you eat does not mean the more fats you will lose. The concept of *calorie in, calorie out* does not apply in the long run. Our body functions way more complex than this mechanism. Converting foods that we eat and the fats in our hips into energy doesn't happen in an instant, but ample time is necessary for this to occur.

Contrary to common knowledge, sugar, in the form of glucose or carbohydrates, is not the only source of energy for us to function efficiently. And skipping meals, even for days, will not lead to death. If you are here to lose the excess fats fast, then you must accept that you need to do more than just reduce your food intake.

Simply put, we must go back to a state on how our ancestors lived their lives before.

With science to back it up, we must accept that *fasting* is an integral part of the human's way of life throughout evolution. This can be further understood by knowing the types of *fuel expenditure* our body uses during different *periods of fasting*. In simpler words, this only means that your energy source will change as days go by without eating. The energy currency in your body is the Adenosine *triphosphate (ATP) molecule*. And it will come from a different energy source, depending on where you are at a given point in time. And yes, glucose is not your only source of energy.

The following are bound to happen on average:

DAY 1: First day without food intake, your body will scrape off all the carbohydrates you have left in your bloodstream, known as your blood glucose, and the remaining ones in your stomach and intestines from your last meal. The energy from glucose is obtained through a process called **glycolysis**.

This will be enough to fuel your daily activity. Note that you will feel hungry, but not the entire day. Instead, you will only feel hungry for about 3-4 times a day, depending on how frequently you take your usual meals. The hunger you will experience is proof of how wired you are to eating at least three meals a day. If you do not give in to the growling sounds of your stomach, it will subside after about an hour. You should not worry about hyperacidity since food is the primary trigger for acid secretions. If you avoid food, including seeing and smelling food, secretion of gastric acids will be suppressed. Your fuel source as of this time is carbohydrates/glucose. Drink some water and take a pinch of salt (or sodium chloride) whenever you feel hungry, a little weak, dizzy or moody, since thirst and hyponatremia (low sodium level in the blood) have the same symptoms as hunger. Each cycle of glycolysis will yield 2 ATP for energy.

DAY 2: At approximately 24-48 hours of fasting, your blood glucose is already depleted. This time, it will tap your glucose stores in the form of glycogen mainly found in your liver. Glycogen is our body's limited carbohydrate reserve. This glycogen will be broken down into glucose through the process of **glycogenolysis**, and the glucose will again undergo glycolysis as it did on the first day. Thus, your fuel source is still mainly carbohydrates, especially if you are not on a low-carb diet to begin with. And depending on the amount of your glycogen stores (about 2,000 kcal on average), or your physical activity, the rate of depletion follows. Note that ketosis, or fat-burning for energy, begins as early as 18 hours after your last carbohydrate-rich meal, and so, energy sources are mixed during this time. You will still feel hungry, but again, only during your usual eating times. Some feel they are hungrier on this day than the previous day, while others feel that the hunger sensation is starting to lessen. Once you can overcome the first 48 hours, chances are, the subsequent days will be easier.

DAY 3: Within 48-72 hours of fasting, you will no longer have extra glucose in your system, (*remember that it is the fuel source that your body has been used to for the longest time*). As of this point, it will tap the next easiest source of energy in your body and create its own glucose. The substrates or *ingredients* will come from fats (the glycerol from triglycerides) and glucogenic amino acids which will come from proteins, mostly exhausting first the misfolded A.K.A "junk" proteins that piled up in the wrong places in your body. If you no longer have those, to some extent, your muscles, but this is rare and should not be cause of worry. I know you might not feel comfortable that the probably little muscles you have will be compromised. Note that it is only very minimal and will not last for long simply because your body, brilliant as it is, knows that it is not sustainable. This process called **gluconeogenesis** or the making of new glucose from your own free triglycerides/fats and proteins, is only an emergency fund, and not designed for long- term use because it will eventually make you weak should it persist. In fact, one may feel he is at his weakest at this point and may already want to give up.

But it is during this time that you must hang on and take some electrolytes, or just water and salt, so your weakness, perceived or otherwise, will be relieved. As they say, rest or even sleep if you must, and listen to your body and not your food-addicted brain. Gluconeogenesis will require 4 ATPs to occur, in order to obtain glucose for glycolysis, that will only yield 2 ATPs. At this point, you can see that this process is not sustainable simply because the net ATP is *negative*, and our body is not wired to self-destruct. Around this time, ketosis is starting to peak. If you set aside the craving, you will see that you have a newfound energy that you might have not experienced before. This is from ketones, an energy fuel coming from fats.

DAY 4 and up: About 72-96 hours of fasting, your body already senses that no food is going to arrive anytime soon. Thus, it will tap its stored energy from your precious vault of fats. Yes, finally, it will use up your fats as the body's new primary energy source in maximum capacity. This process is called **lypolysis**, which simply means breakdown of lipids. As of this point, the real and major fat breakdown occurs.

Fat's usable energy form is called ketone bodies and it can start to occur after about *18 hours of fasting* and becomes more pronounced the longer the person *fasts*. This is also known as **Ketosis** or the shifting of energy stores from glucose to ketones. Ketone bodies are very energy-dense molecules, wherein one ketone body will yield 22 ATPs. This explains why there are so many testimonials saying that after days of fasting, they felt a sense of increased strength and energy and even improved mental prowess. Not known to many, **Ketones** are the preferred fuel source by many organs, including the brain, and once adapted in *Ketosis,* even the other organs like muscles can now utilize ketones as an efficient energy source. For some, there is this stage of *Keto Flu*, wherein one experiences signs and symptoms of flu without having an actual flu because the body is still adjusting. This is because our body is not used to using ketones as a fuel, and simply because, just like every other regular human, we've never really and truly *fasted* our entire lives. But on days 4 to 5, hunger is already at minimum, though you can still feel it occurring the same time on the previous days, but this time, it won't bother you anymore because the hunger hormone *Ghrelin* is already declining, as proven in studies on supervised prolonged fasts.

Again, note that there may be an overlap among these biochemical processes. Some studies indicate that ketosis starts to occur as early as 12 hours of fasting, with heavy ketosis occurring at 18 hours.

For some people and even other fellow doctors, the mere mention of ketosis already signifies a big red flag. This is because basic biochemistry books in medical school discuss ketosis very briefly and it is always subsequently alongside starvation and diabetic *ketoacidosis,* which can be fatal.

However, they failed to emphasize that ketoacidosis occurs when there is a persistently high level of blood glucose, together with high level of ketones among diabetic patients, whose food intake is largely composed of sugar and/or absence of insulin to regulate the sugar within the bloodstream. However, for those who are non-diabetics, fasting will follow the normal transition of fuel source (carbohydrate to fats), thus blood glucose will decrease and only ketones will increase to a nutritional level, where weight loss, and most importantly, healing, are achieved. Blood ketone levels for steady weight loss is at approximately 1.0-3.0 mmol/L when doing short extended fasts, whereas heavy ketosis and greater weight loss effects are achieved during prolonged extended fast, and even this seldom reach more than 5.0 mmol/L. Even at more elevated levels, it will NOT cause acidosis because ketones are naturally produced when fat burning mechanism ensues. The dangerous level of ketoacidosis is at 10 mmol/L and occurs together with elevated blood glucose as a complication of type 1 diabetes. This level is not seen among those with normal pancreas because of the counter regulatory mechanism of producing insulin in response to ketones that are going beyond the nutritional ketosis level of 5mg/dL.

Thus, once fully adapted at the level of nutritional ketosis, your blood sugar and insulin are at a stable level and in the lower range of normal, where they should always be.

According to *Loren Lockman*, advocate of water fasting and one who supervised thousands of long-term extended fasts, an average person has the capacity to do a safe water-only fasting for up to six weeks. That if you have fat stores and your body fat percentage does not go down below 5-12%, you can live with energy coming from ketones & gluconeogenesis only. The longest recorded fast in a medical journal is 382 days and the subject stopped when he finally reached his ideal weight. He sustained the weight loss and had normal BMI throughout his remaining life.

I know at this point you might have doubts, especially with your capacity to do it. I know because I had doubts too, because in my 30 years of existence prior to discovering the wonders of fasting, I have never had a day where I had not had any food.

But after thorough research and scientific build-up of confidence, I trusted the process. I decided to put my faith in nature, knowing that fasting has been an integral part of human evolution and it is a practice of almost all religions from time immemorial. I started my first five days of water-only fasting, relying not on how I was raised, or what the media advertisements say, but on the evolutionary perspective's scientific confidence as to why fasting can be done safely and smoothly. I trusted the fact that because our genes have been through thousands of years of experience, it enabled our body to sustain it. Surprisingly, not known to many, our body is more adapted to scarcity than gluttony.

And as I went through the fasting days, with psychological turmoil going on inside my head, I found solace, knowing that regular extended fasting has been a way of life for millions of people all over the world. Miles and miles away from where I live, people are connecting and supporting each other during extended fasting. Hundreds of blogs and videos discuss the benefits of fasting and even documenting their daily update during an active fast.

I successfully completed a 5-day water-only fast while continuously and properly working in the hospital, doing my usual ward to emergency department duties and surgeries. From the food indulger that I was, I became liberated from food dependency. From seeking food all the time, my mental strength has never been better. I felt like a totally different person, that I have achieved a certain level of elation that nothing else can give. It is a level of confidence and empowerment that only you can give yourself. If I can do it, I know you can too.

Imagine a few days of psychological exercise, in exchange for finally attaining the body and health you've always been dreaming of.

Fasting can be done in various schedules and lengths. After more than 50 months since I started extended fasting, I did multiple long fasts of five to 14 days with no food intake, something that I did for specific medical, academic, and spiritual purposes, with the right preparation, place of rest, vital signs and laboratory monitoring, and mindset.

With proper guidance from this book, anybody can do it at their own convenience and keep on doing it until they reach their ideal body image or as long as their body tells them when they should do it. And you do not need to do the whole three days or more, not even a full 24 hours because there are smoother ways to reach ketosis, other than engaging in a prolonged fast.

Want it and it will be yours. Trust that it can be done. Write down your goals and why you want to achieve that. Focus on that goal and let it be your fuel to give *fasting* a try. There is nothing else better than you yourself in control of both your body and your mind.

STAGES of FASTING Summary

Day 1: Fuel source is mostly from Blood Sugar/ Glucose, hunger pangs are severe, this can lead to lowering of your blood sugar and water loss as well. Mild ketosis starts to occur.

Day 2: Fuel Source is still mostly from Sugar/Glucose coming from the storage form Glycogen mostly from the liver, hunger may decrease but may be worse for some, this will deplete the glycogen in the liver. This is also the beginning of heavier ketosis.

Day 3: Fuel source is mostly from Ketones, and this is when keto flu, keto breath, and fruity urine can occur from *ketone dumping* because the majority of the organs are not yet fully ketone-adapted. The body is producing more ketones than the organs have learned to accept yet. The need for glucose by the red blood cells and some obligate glucose-dependent cells are supplemented by gluconeogenesis made from the breakdown of fats (triglycerides) and proteins. This is the start of significant fat loss.

Day 4 and beyond: Major fuel source is now ketones, which can come from your fat stores, hunger is at its lowest, and this is the stage where pure fat loss occurs and blood sugar and insulin are low normal, but stable. Do the Salt Fix, or intake of pinch of salt and water, whenever you feel temporary hunger, thirst, headache, or even irritability.

CHAPTER 3

Why Meal Timing Matters
Recognizing "when to eat" is the key

> *"If anything is worth doing,*
> *do it with all your heart."*
>
> -Buddha

Fasting is essential to strike a balance in one's way of life. However, it is not sustainable for you to keep on fasting all throughout, because then, no balance shall result. This is the point where we answer the question: when should we really eat for us to get back the eating equilibrium our generation has lost?

And the answer is "No, it's not your usual breakfast-lunch-dinner routine. Nor is it being the kindergarten's *breakfast - morning snacks - lunch - afternoon snacks - dinner - bedtime milk time"* routine. When to eat, it should be something instinctive. Like the animals in the wild, we humans are supposed to eat only when we are hungry and stop eating when we are full. Following these instincts, no one should become overweight (except for special natural occurrences like pregnancy and growth of a child). So, if this is the case, when did we go wrong? Why is obesity starting to become a worldwide pandemic, especially among the resource-sufficient parts of the world?

Unfortunately, this comes down with nature versus nurture. For our generation, unfortunately, nurture took reign.

Remember when you were forced to eat as a child even when you don't want to? Or when you were forced to stay at the dinner table until you finished everything your mother put on your plate? And no, it's not your parent's fault. Because like almost everyone on this planet plagued by the marketing strategies of the multi-billion food industry, parents too are fooled by statements like, *"Breakfast is the most important meal of the day"* or *"Always be ready, never go hungry"* schemes.

As it turned out, those hard-to-put-on-breakfast-table kids, are the ones we should follow. Those kids are listening and responding to their instincts, that they should eat only when their bodies are already in need of nutrition, and they stop when they've had enough. However, with the constant *reward-punishment parenting model* we adults unknowingly follow, plus the undeniable pleasure from sweets and simple sugars, those instincts are eventually lost. By nature, hunger hormone *Ghrelin* increases when your body is truly hungry (as in lacking energy and resources to finish a certain task). However, over time, *Ghrelin* increases simply because the body is used to receiving food during specific times of the day, despite the abundant food storage in our bodies in the form of fats.

Studies show that during a 24-hour monitoring, *Ghrelin* increases in response to the usual eating time and corresponds to the hunger pangs a person is experiencing when not giving in to the hunger sensation occasioned by this hormone. It is important to note that over time, contrary to common knowledge, *one does not get hungrier as time passes*. Instead, the sense of hunger will pass after about an hour and will only recur during the next mealtime, with just about the same or even lesser hunger sensation than before, indicating a declining *Ghrelin* level as the days of fasting go by. If one eats, especially when eating a low carbohydrate diet with adequate protein and high in healthy fats, the fullness hormone *Leptin* increases, and this signals your brain to stop eating. This is the reason why animals in the wild don't become obese because there is a balance between *Ghrelin* and *Leptin* in their body and they respond to it accordingly.

So, how can we re-establish a balanced and well-functioning *Ghrelin* and *Leptin*?

Simple, just unlearn what you have learned. That is, intentionally disrupting the eating pattern you've been used to your whole life.

By not responding to the urge to eat just because it's 7:00 AM, and to consciously refuse food intake when you know you still have a lot of fats in your body. Yes, in a word, what you need to do is *fast*. To regain your instinctive drive, you can slowly reset your body to its natural state.

Fasting is the key to **appetite correction** or the reestablishment of balance between *Leptin and Ghrelin hormones*. There's a rapid way, and there's a smooth slow way. But if significant weight loss is your goal, then, you can go for the highway - in this case, scheduled fasting.

CHAPTER 4

The Basics of Fasting

Must-knows every future faster needs

> *"The secret of change is to focus all of your energy, not on fighting the old, but on building the new."*
>
> -Socrates

To embark on the highway option, the first thing you need to do is to know what fasting really means. As described by the founder of Intensive Dietary Management and Nephrologist Dr. Jason Fung, in his books: The Obesity Code (with co-author Jim Moore), The Complete Guide to Fasting, it is clearly explained that fasting is not synonymous to starvation. Fasting is the voluntary non-consumption or omission of calorie-containing food and beverages.

Whereas, starvation, is the involuntary absence or negation of food intake, despite the person's protest or natural need for food sustenance. Although they may initially affect one's physical aspects similarly, the large difference is on the emotional and psychological impact each has. With starvation, detrimental effects of feeling of vulnerability and helplessness can ensue.

Whereas in fasting, the person is in control, he is totally in charge, empowering him for every hour endured knowing that one can break it anytime as desired. Fasting has impacted those who practice it, not just physically, but also mentally and spiritually and in a good way.

There are so many fasting schedules available for everyone (*daily or weekly bases*) and you can study them and see which fasting routine can work for you.

As hard to believe as it may seem, the struggle in fasting is about 95% psychological and only 5% physical (for those with excess fats to lose).

In general, fasting is considered *fasting* if you have not taken any calorie containing food and drinks for at least 12 hours.

Studies show that after 12 hours, ketosis or breakdown of fats already starts. And by the 18th hour, you are already in heavy ketosis, where a large part of your energy is coming from ketones. If you extend it to 24 hours, other health-enhancing benefits occur, but the most important of which, as of this point, is the commencement of the burning of heavily guarded and highly stubborn stored fats. These fats may not be that obvious for some because it could be hidden inside our bellies, covering our organs, or even infiltrating it like in Fatty Liver. The longer you fast, the more stubborn fats you lose. It's that simple.

During your fasting period, you can consume as much water, natural tea leaves, or black coffee with salt and electrolytes you want, especially if you fast for less than 24 hours. This is called a *Clean Fast* and is something that I advocate whenever I engage in a daily intermittent fast or short-term extended fast. You should always be mindful of how your body responds and you should keep yourself hydrated, including electrolytes, especially salt.

That is why prolonged fasting can sometimes lead to electrolyte-imbalance in certain people, especially that a significant number of electrolytes are continuously eliminated in urine if these are not replenished accordingly. Thus, to avoid such occurrence, consumption of electrolyte and micronutrient-containing liquids are allowed, as long as it does not contain any calories, nor it has a sweet taste like artificial sweeteners. Only zero-calorie liquids that contain electrolytes may be consumed, especially during prolonged fasting. Examples include water, coffee, tea, filtered vinegar, best with salt and electrolytes.

As identified by Gin Stephen's book *"Delay, Don't Deny"*, any additional consumption is already classified as *dirty fasting* and such is not advisable because even if you do not eat any solid foods, consumption of any calorie-containing liquid or even zero-calorie foodstuff having a sweet taste (like the diet sodas and juices) can already stop the healing processes seen in *Clean Fasting*.

On another note, according to *Dr. Jason Fung*, during an *extended fast of more than 24 hours,* certain amounts of good fats may be incorporated, in addition to the previously stated allowed fluids, whenever one feels weak but doesn't want to break the fast. These include coconut oil, heavy cream, medium-chain triglyceride oil, or bone and vegetable broth. These additions will not jeopardize your fasting state in terms of fat-burning because these fat-rich substances will still chemically mimic fasting, or *fat-fasting*, thus, will not kick one out of ketosis. Personally, I recommend doing an initial dry fast, followed by *clean water-only fasting* with salt as needed, for as long as you can to maximize not just fat-burning, but more so on healing. If there comes a point of feeling weak, one can consume salt water, potassium, and magnesium supplements since those are the electrolytes that are frequently lost. If the weakness persists and continues to worsen, *fat-fasting* may be done by consuming any pure natural fats or bone broth. Note that consuming anything with flavor, even if it has zero calories, can trigger hunger more, thus you must be careful with what you choose to consume during your fasting. Details on the fluids you can take during fasting will be discussed in the next chapter.

As previously discussed, each stage of fasting will have a different effect on one's body. This is the best time to review the summary of stages of fasting and the corresponding fuel source being utilized, as first seen in Chapter 2.

CHAPTER 5

Dry Fasting, Wet Fasting & Fluids
Water is the best of all

"The noblest of all studies is the study of what man is and of what life he should live."

-Plato

Of all fluids there is, the most important, luckily the cheapest, water. Clean, natural water is ideal, but any unflavored water may also do.

But before we discuss the fluids, let's first tackle one of the major improvements of this edition: the underrated Dry Fasting (DF).

In the first edition, I was very dismissive of the idea of DF. This is primarily because, as a newbie in the world of fasting, and as someone who is trying to open the average person into this once unpopular concept, DF just seemed too much. But now, with significant change in the mindset of this social media era, just less than four years before the first edition was published, almost everyone now has heard of Intermittent Fasting. Thus, I feel the reader of this second edition is now more open to this yet another seemingly counterproductive behavior.

Dry fasting for me is the purest form of fasting. This is done without consuming food and all forms of externally obtained fluids, making it prudent to discuss this, and I will try to do so as briefly as I can.

For practitioners of DF, it is further divided into two. (1) Soft DF is when contact with water is allowed as long as it is not consumed *per Orem* or taken in the gut. Examples would include brushing one's teeth, taking a bath, or douching any cavity in the body. Based on physiologic outcomes, this is the more preferred method between the two as it gives some hydration to the skin without jeopardizing the metabolic benefits of DF. (2) Hard DF, on the other hand, is total abstinence of any contact with water, some even as extreme as not swallowing their own saliva. Based on testimonies of people who did it, there is greater impact when it comes to their psyche, especially for those who are doing it for spiritual and non-physiologic reasons (*Personally, I have only been an avid practitioner of Soft DF*).

As much as it is a common knowledge that three days without water can lead to death, the case is simply not true, or at least, not for me and the other people I personally know, and those I know online who have undergone DF for as long as 21 days.

If this is the first time that you've heard about DF, it might be surprising for you to realize that the scientific explanation is quite simple.

Yes, our body cannot function without water. That is the basic premise of those who are saying that we cannot live for weeks without it. And yes, that is true. But what they missed is the fact that our body can produce water. Yes, and that is a fact. The purest and cleanest form of water known to man (*and the rest of the animal kingdom*) is the one endogenously made by his own cells; this is called Metabolic Water. In other words, this makes water technically non-essential because we can create it from scratch inside our own body. Per gram of fat metabolized or burned, is said to produce about 1.1 ml of metabolic water, whereas per gram of carbohydrates will yield 0.6 ml and proteins at 0.4 ml. Among the three macronutrients, it is only the burning of fats that can be a prolonged source of Metabolic Water in times of complete drought, because our body lacks the capacity of storing large reserves of carbohydrates, while protein metabolism will have metabolites that is needing roughly the same amount of water, for it to be safely excreted as urea and not be retained as ammonia. This makes both protein and carbohydrates an inefficient source of Metabolic Water.

Knowing those basics, one can now understand that with DF, a person can live without drinking water provided he still has enough fat reserves that can be burned for the body's need of Metabolic Water.

We already know that general fasting burns fats for energy. But when it is Dry Fasting, fat burning is accelerated because the body's motivation to do so is now doubled: first is the need for extra energy, and now, the need for water, which is a far greater trigger than the former.

To give you an example, let's do a little math with the following values:

1 gram of fat will yield:
    9 Kcal
    1.1ml of Metabolic Water

If a person needs 1,800 Kcal a day, he can simply burn 200 grams of fat mass to do that. (1,800 Kcal/ 9 Kcal/gram = 200 grams)

However, if a person needs 1,000 ml of water, he must burn at least 900 grams of fats to produce that. (1,000 ml/ 1.1 ml/gram = 909 grams)

This comparison makes the fat burning 4.5x greater for the formation of Metabolic Water than Energy production.

That is the reason why DF is said to be at least 3x more effective than Wet Fasting (WF) when it comes to fat burning. Note, though, that this is not an equation that can be deduced perfectly from person to person since there are other intricate biochemical steps that involve subtraction and addition in the metabolic pathway. Instead, this just serves as a rough estimate showing the disparity between the two.

Scientific studies on humans while performing DF is still limited to 12-24 hours only. The most widely known practitioners of DF are the ones practicing *Ramadan,* approximately 14 hours daily for about a month annually. Thus, I cannot specifically provide any direct support in promoting DF that is longer than that.

So, in a gist, DF will provide the benefits similar to regular wet or water fasting but with accelerated results. Top 6 of those are the following:

1. Weight loss, especially fat loss
2. Lowered inflammation in the majority of forms through excretion of harmful metabolites that accumulated in the various tissues for years.
3. Increase BDNF, increases Serotonin that it makes the person feel elated and at the same time improves cognitive function.
4. Prevent osteoporosis and at the same time skin and other soft tissue rejuvenation through stem cell activation & autophagy.
5. Lowers blood sugar and insulin levels.
6. Improves cholesterol profile when done regularly.

However, as excited as you might be in DF, these seven things should always be in mind:

1. Side effects of regular IF can be heightened when it is a DF, thus one should always be prepared.
2. If considered, one should ease in slowly starting with as little as 7-8 hours during sleeping and slowly increase to

facilitate adaptation.
3. Breaking the fast in DF needs an even slower process as the risk for rebound water retention and Refeeding Syndrome is greater.
4. DF is done for a specific kind of healing. It shouldn't be done for weight loss purposes alone as this is a tricky tool for that.
5. If done daily, then 12-16 hours is already enough. If longer than that, it should be scheduled accordingly to avoid disruption of one's metabolism.
6. Doing DF should not be treated as a ticket to eat junk during one's eating window.
7. To sustain the benefits of DF, a proper refeeding is equally important and should contain a good amount of quality proteins, essential micronutrients, and other natural foods that will not trigger insulin spike.

Contrary to DF, *Wet Fasting* is a type of fasting that allows one to consume fluids while abstaining from solid food. Variations include *Pure Water Fast*, *Clean Fast* with Electrolytes and other non-calorie containing fluids, and lastly, *Fat Fast* including intake of fatty substance and other fluids with no significant amount of macronutrients that do not break ketosis. Other kinds of "fast" not mentioned here, like egg and banana fast, no meat fast, oatmeal fast, and other forms of food restriction that does doesn't lower the insulin response and do not lead into full ketosis, are not considered as true metabolic fasting, but just considered as a low-calorie kind of intake.

Water-only fast has proven to be good if one cannot do DF with a central aim of fat loss because intake of anything that needs metabolizing will take up energy from your body. With water-only fast, a person is practicing his body to function at its optimum with little to no sustenance, except water. Without any flavor that passes through your gut, you can provide rest to your bowels, pancreas, and the rest of your gastrointestinal tract. Upon introduction to your system, without any intake of nutrients, this will enable the very basic processes of converting glucose, glycogen and fats into energy that may be used for daily tasks and for facilitating fat loss.

During fasting it is very important that you take time to listen to your body. Identify temporary hunger pangs due to routine eating time versus hunger due to true nutrient deficiency. Always have water in hand as it is important to be kept hydrated. However, it is also equally important not to "over hydrate" by consuming water way more than what you need. overhydration may be suspected if you experience frequent urination and is experienced almost immediately after water intake with the same or more amount than you took, followed by episodes of worsening muscle weakness. This is because water and sodium go together as they are eliminated in your urine. By Water-fast, intake is generally not similar to 8-10 glasses of water as you do on a normal day. Instead, just small sips when thirst is unbearable can be done. Otherwise, over intake of water without a balance of electrolytes can lead to hypotonic dehydration.

As a result, you will become sodium-deficient or *hyponatremic* which will manifest as weakness, easy fatigability, headache, and light-headedness. But, if you listen to your body carefully, and by drinking sips of water, little by little only, whenever you feel thirsty or hungry, and avoid gulping liters in one setting, one can eliminate the risk of *overhydration* complications.

However, if such symptoms still occur, it is at this point that you can add non-caloric substance to your water that will not break your fast and will not aggravate hunger but can help sustain your fasting commitment. These are essential electrolytes that get deficient during prolonged fasting with normal day to day activity. In my case, I find that a teaspoon of vinegar, mixed with a pinch of salt and diluted with two tablespoons of water, suppresses my appetite and gives me an energy boost from sodium replacement. Note that this is just a personal preference since I cannot seem to tolerate intake of salty water alone. In times where I cannot have that concoction, I take rock salts directly instead.

I have been doing countless Extended Fasting (EFs) while doing my regular routine, but it is important to note that for safety, especially for beginners, there are fasting advocates who advise total bed rest during this period.

Only a few influencers promote extended WF without any supplements, however, after years of personal research and experience, I find this dangerous because it puts the body easily at risk of electrolyte imbalance that can have serious clinical implications.

When fasting for 1-2 weeks, electrolytes like sodium, magnesium, and to some extent, potassium supplements, will be needed. However, for longer fasts, additional supplementation of calcium, chloride and phosphorus may be necessary to avoid risk of *re-feeding syndrome.*

Below is a list of common electrolytes important in fasting and its corresponding symptoms of deficiency:

    1. Sodium Chloride (Salt)

Sodium as the basic chemical component of salt is the most abundant extracellular electrolyte in our body. It is one of the most common components for humans to perform regular functions, and its most important organ regulator is our kidneys. When one has more sodium, kidneys just simply eliminate it through urine and when the same is depleting, the kidney will try to keep whatever amount it can save before urinating. However, it is not that easy to perfect the optimum water intake, and to teach kidneys to readily save all the salts you have during your first few days of fasting. Thus, to slowly introduce the transition, you can prepare and infuse your body with homemade salt water, and take sips when necessary. (*Again, I find that mixing salt, water and vinegar is more palatable than salt and water alone.*)

You will be amazed that you can immediately feel some improvement on your strength, headache, or usual early fast symptoms after you take a sip. The more organic the salt, the better it is. Good reviews were handed to pink Himalayan salts, but I find any salt to perform the job just as fine. Of course, pure, organic and natural salt is ideal. To make your own concoction, just take 1 tablespoon of salt and mix it with 50-500 ml of water. Whatever amount left that day should be discarded and make another one for the next day. Or, simply have a pinch of salt to your tongue and flush it with a sip or gulp of water as needed. Signs and symptoms of low sodium or *hyponatremia* include muscle cramps, loss of appetite, nausea, headache, and dizziness. These symptoms are often attributed to *hypoglycemia* or low blood sugar, but often, it is just due to low salt in the body. Thus, if this happens, take some and see the improvements after. This is also called *"The Salt Fix"* by Dr. Nico Dinicolantonio.

2. Magnesium

While magnesium is commonly disregarded, it is in fact very important in processes that involve electrical impulses in the body, particularly in the muscles, nerves, and heart. Symptoms of deficiency will include muscular cramps and spasms, difficulty to concentrate, and palpitations. Generally, we have an abundance of Magnesium stores in our bones. However, its release may not be as readily as we need it and the need for supplement varies greatly from person to person. During the first 1-3 days, seldom does hypomagnesemia occur. But as your fasting progresses and you start to feel these symptoms to occur, you can consider taking in magnesium supplements at 200 to 400 mg per day. Personally, I only noticed symptoms of muscle cramps on the 10th day of water only fasting. Again, this varies greatly, especially on individual's bodily stores.

3. Potassium

This is the most important intracellular ion in the body. It functions hand in hand with sodium. And since sodium loss is expected especially during the early phase of fasting, potassium loss or *hypokalemia* can also ensue.

Symptoms of hypokalemia can include muscle weakness, blood pressure changes, palpitations, muscle cramps, and in severe cases, mental confusion. Thus, it is optimum to have potassium supplements in handy when engaging in extended fast (>5-7 days). The amount you need will depend on your physical activity. If you are an athlete or doing heavy physical labor, you can consider taking in a little more than the recommended daily allowance of 1,500 up to 3,500 mg for the average adult. However, for those that are not engaging in strenuous activities, potassium is seldom required even in extended fasts of more than 5-7 days, provided that sodium and water intake is optimum.

Aside from those, there are also other electrolytes that are needed in small amounts but seldom cause problems, unless you are very physically active or doing resistance training or already have signs of osteoporosis. These include calcium, chloride (already part of salt as sodium chloride), bicarbonate, phosphorus and phosphates.

However, if EF is considered while one is still young without co-morbidities and are not engaging in laborious routine, he/she can proceed without taking much of the latter supplements. On the other hand, if a person feels the need for them, further readings are suggested.

Remember, electrolyte deficiency is the most common cause of **Keto Flu**, and a resultant termination of fasting. It is of great importance to prepare and properly equip yourself prior to embarking on an extended fast in order for you to be fully prepared and attain success in this journey.

Other than electrolytes, some non-caloric additions can improve the fasting experience. This is considered a clean fast.

Coffee - whether with or without caffeine, as long as there is no sugar or cream, is a good addition to your water. It boosts your metabolism and is a great option for those who are avid coffee drinkers. For those who are not used to taking in black coffee (i.e. no sugar or cream), you can start taking it as light as possible and slowly increase the strength to suit your taste. Note though that it may exacerbate dehydration because of caffeine's diuretic effect in the kidneys and can worsen the temporary sleep disturbance that is usually experienced during EF. Even decaffeinated coffee still contains about 25-33% caffeine compared to regular coffee.

Tea - any organic tea leaves is okay to add flavor to your water, in addition to the inherent properties of individual teas (i.e. green tea's appetite suppression, calming effect of chamomile, caffeine-fix of black teas). Again, some effects of caffeine may be noted in teas containing it.

Zero calorie spices like cinnamon, ginger or turmeric are also welcome, however, carefully consider prior to adding these since flavor can instantly trigger appetite and subsequent hunger sensation might result.

Judicious amount of water with electrolytes is the best fluid you can take in achieving functional, energy- sufficient fasting days. Fasting without any fluids, which is called dry fasting, should be done with lots of caution and consideration as detailed above.

When engaging in your first extended fast, I suggest keeping it as clean as possible, as whatever length of time you clock in, is already a lifetime's worth of personal achievement that you can take pride and make reference to. For instance, a week-long water-only fasting, is a bragging record and a motivational reference for your future self; that if you can do it that one time, surely you can do it again and can readily take on any other less challenging tasks, and mind you, there are too many less challenging tasks than saying no to any amount and any type of food for days.

On the other hand, below are the fluids you can consume while on Fat Fasting (*previously termed as Dirty Fasting*), a variation advised by Dr. Jason Fung in his book entitled, *The Obesity Code and The Complete Guide to Fasting.* These fluids have high fat and nutrient contents, that even if you are truly already breaking your fast by consuming calories, "biochemically" you are still fasting because you would be continuously utilizing fats/ketones, thus, you are not getting out of ketosis stage or the fat burning stage and you can proceed with the burning of your own body's fat stores thereafter.

1. Vegetable Broth - the soup from cooked vegetables and spices. Strain the vegetables and sip the soup only. May contain a trace amount of calories from carbohydrates and/or plant proteins, but a good source of electrolytes and some micronutrients to quench your thirst and to some extent, hunger. *(Fat Fast)*

2. Bone Broth - the soup from boiled meat, preferably with bones. Strain and sip especially when feeling weak during extended fasting. *(Fat Fast)*

3. Bulletproof coffee - one cup of black coffee and froth with 1 tablespoon of fats like coconut oil, medium chain triglyceride (MCT) oil, whole milk, butter, heavy cream, or cinnamon for flavor. Limit to only 1-2 servings per day. *(Fat Fast)*

4. Water with natural filtered vinegar (apple cider or pure coconut vinegar) - shown to have good effects on appetite suppression and epigastric pain from stomach acid secretions. Mix one tablespoon of vinegar, with or without salt, in 100 ml of water. Dilute as tolerated. *(Clean Fast)*

5. Water with lemon and lime or fruit slices without consuming these. The citrus extracts will add flavor to water but this may contain some sugar. May contain some trace calories but not significant to halt ketosis *(Fat Fast)*

To recap, water with electrolytes is considered clean fasting. Other zero-calorie and non-sweet fluids like black coffee, tea, and vinegar can be taken in a clean fast.

Personally, I take pleasure in pure, organic zero calorie vinegar (coconut or apple cider) mixed with salt and water, which is a very good source of electrolytes and an effective appetite suppressant when fasting. I understand that many are aversive to vinegar, thus, feel free to experiment on items you can mix and match without breaking your clean fast. Some even put salt in their coffee, and yes, it removes its bitterness and replaces it with salty taste, so, you can also personalize your own.

Clean fasting should be advocated for daily intermittent fast (IF) after sleeping on a Dry Fast (meaning, you do not need to take water in the middle of your sleep), and as long as you can during extended fast (EF). Other fluid additions should only be considered when doing the latter. Differentiation between IF and EF will be discussed in the succeeding chapters.

Again, I am putting emphasis on these types of fasting in descending order in a matter of purity and priority when fasting.

First is the short-term Dry Fasting, second is the Clean Fasting *(water plus minimal salt)*. Once I already feel weak, too bored that I want to end my fasting, or with signs of electrolyte imbalance, I will proceed with a *clean fast*, wherein black coffee, tea, and other electrolytes can be added. Lastly, when engaging in a fast of more than three days, I allow myself to have *fat fasting* when I can no longer stick to clean fasting for whatever reason, and if I cannot sustain it, I then decide to break the fast.

A special note on Dry Fasting:

During the last 4 years since I've started a fasting lifestyle, I have completed multiple 3-4 days of DF and the longest was seven days of Soft DF, followed by another seven days of WF. I have done it for experimentation and with medical preparation, and I do not recommend anyone doing it on their own. That schedule is called Phoenix Protocol that is said to be a variation of what few Russians doctors employ to promote longevity and is said to extend lifespan up to 25 years when done 1-4x a year. For interested readers, you may explore this topic more and do so with caution.

CHAPTER 6

Who Can Fast

"Our souls need fasting as much as our bodies need food."

-Islamic Proverb

As we are all descendants of humanity, and so, it is just a given that anybody can actually fast. In fact, everybody has fasted many times in the past without knowing it. The daily gap between your dinner and breakfast the following day is already *fasting*, thus the term "breakfast", or breaking a fast.

Noteworthy though, benefits are seen when fasting is extended to a minimum of 12 hours, just enough to rid your bloodstream of the extra sugars you've had the previous day. Weight loss from fat burning and subsequent ketosis, starts to significantly kick in after the 16th hour and can be slowly extended to as long as tolerated.

Any adult who wants to lose weight, with the right mental understanding of the risks and benefits of fasting, can engage in such. Anybody who is physically able without any known illness, not taking any medications and are desirous of improving their overall health, are the best people to start this journey.

If you have illnesses and/or symptoms related to any lifestyle diseases such as obesity, chronic pain, diabetes, hypertension, and elevated cholesterol, you can still engage in fasting provided, ideally, you have proper guidance from your trusted physician.

The latter subgroup can benefit the most from fasting, and studies show that these lifestyle diseases even have the potential to be reversed. This claim was supported by my own patients and the hundreds of thousands members of our Low Carb and Fasting online community who are sharing their success stories. Although there are a lot of success stories from those who did it on their own, *DIY style*, it is highly advised that thorough consideration, research, and preparation should be done first, before engaging in any type of extended fasting.

Although in general, daily and short intermittent fasting can be smoothly executed by those with maintenance medications and in need of frequent monitoring, any form of extended fast must be done with guidance or under the direct supervision of healthcare professionals since individual medical history and response vary from person to person.

For those with no known serious illness and without symptoms suggesting such, generally healthy, young or otherwise, and have extra fats to manage or needed reduction, then it is best to start immediately while risks are minimal, and benefits are at best. Incorporation of at least 12 hours of daily IF can already do so much, for healing, disease prevention and health preservation, especially when one is eating clean during his eating window. This will be discussed further in the next chapters.

CHAPTER 7

Who Cannot Fast

"I'm not telling you it's going to be easy, I am telling you it's going to be worth it."

-Anonymous

Fasting, especially extended fasting, is not recommended among limited groups of individuals belonging in these subgroups:

Growing children

As they are still in their developmental years, children are prohibited from engaging in intentional and extended fasts. The nutrients from food are essential for them to reach developmental maturity. For very young children, their peripheral fats are essential in heat regulation to avoid hypothermia, thus, fat loss during this period is strongly discouraged. They, however, can benefit from eating in moderation and meal timing that is not dictated by routine, but by their instinctive and nutritional bodily needs. In simpler words, there is no need to force children to eat when they do not have the appetite. However, responsible adults should always have real, nutrient-dense foods available for the kids to eat should they feel the need for it. *Ad libitum*, or to eat as needed, is a better approach and best during breastfeeding years, so their natural appetite won't get disrupted. (*A notable exemption for this approach includes children born with genetic, congenital, or acquired disease affecting the appetite regulator in the brain, leading to insatiable hunger. For these few and unfortunate group, professional help is necessary. Good thing, most eating problems in children are manageable, but should start first with elimination of ultra-processed foods in their daily meals.*)

Pregnant and Breastfeeding Women

A special note on those exclusively breastfeeding infants less than 4-6 months old, this is among the most established occurrence in nature, where weight gain is expected and encouraged, as this ensures the proper development of the offspring. Reproduction is a major driver of nature, and it is prioritized above all.

Intentional and prolonged fasting may jeopardize both the health of the baby and the mother; and when nature is forced to choose, the latter is likely to be sacrificed. Thus, the best approach for these women is to eat food that will nourish the child, and at the same time provide for her own, to avoid malnutrition. Note though that this can be abused. That is, some take this time to overeat beyond their needs, thus resulting in serious metabolic problems like gestational diabetes, hypertension, and eclampsia.

A good way to avoid such is by consuming real foods like meat, eggs, fish, certain vegetables, and root crops in a mindful manner to avoid overfeeding.

Although there are a lot of illnesses that can be benefited by fasting, an educated and informed approach should be done before deciding on anything that can possibly put one in danger.

Certain medications affect metabolism in an erratic way, and these are discussed in detail in the second book of this series, *Perfect At Last: Health*, because there is logic to the saying "Better safe than sorry."

Other subgroups that need precaution are as follows:

Comorbidities & Medications

Those on prescription medications and with diagnosed diseases, including those who are currently diagnosed with any medical or psychiatric conditions, are warned not to engage in fasting without prior consultation with their respective physicians. Those with Type 1 Diabetes and other types of Diabetes Mellitus who are taking anti-hyperglycemic medications should be monitored closely for dose adjustments of insulin injection, possible removal, or reduction of other oral medications, to avoid a lethal hypoglycemic episode.

Ulcers

Those with known hyperacidity or predisposed to having stomach ulcers should also be cautioned. Although there are a number of factors that contribute to ulcer formation, an active ulcer or gastritis are sometimes aggravated by fasting, especially if done abruptly without correction of food intake first. Proper treatment of hyperacidity or related illness, like gastroesophageal reflux disease (GERD), and knowledge on how to counter the risk during fasting should be obtained first, prior to considering this course. One approach I find effective is to not think of fasting first, but improve the dietary habits by consuming foods in our Safe List, downloadable at www.jgrtanmd.com or can be found online using a #JGCRojoFoodList, a non-inflammatory diet usually facilitates natural healing of ulcers and gastritis. Once healed, short IF can be started without discomfort.

Syncope & Hyperactive Parasympathetic Response

Those with a history of fainting spells are also warned. Fainting has a lot of possible causes, but the common ones include hypoglycemia, orthostatic hypotension or decrease in blood pressure from sudden positional changes and heightened parasympathetic response in times of extreme stress. Appropriate investigation must be done first prior to fasting as this can trigger that and a risk for trauma increases.

Malnourishment

Those who are undernourished or in cachexia, severe malnutrition such as kwashiorkor and marasmus, as often seen in children in areas with famine, can also be seen in adults. Cachexia manifested by being severely underweight and with muscle wasting, usually from chronic illnesses and late-stage diseases, are contraindicated to undergo fasting.

Eating Disorders

Those with eating disorders, especially those diagnosed with anorexia, are advised against fasting. Certain eating disorders that can benefit from true weight loss should consider doing so only under direct supervision of a professional to help deal with the psychological issues underlying this behavior.

Other specific conditions not mentioned here, or a strong sense of repulsion against fasting, can serve as contraindication to fast. In that case, kindly consult with your trusted physician first should you have doubts whether you can fast or not.

CHAPTER 8

Extended Fasting

"Everyone can perform magic, everyone can reach his goals, if he is able to think, if he is able to wait, if he is able to fast."

— Herman Hesse

No solid food intake for more than 24 hours is already considered an extended fast (EF). There are multiple variations of fasting that are expounded on the books written by Dr. Jason Fung and Gin Stephen, but for the sake of efficient fat loss for better health, I believe that the most natural way is through a scheduled and timely EF of at least 3-5 days mimicking how our hunter and gatherer ancestors did before.

But do not get me wrong, I am not saying you should do it, but it is an idea that stemmed from our evolution that I believe every human should be aware of.

Although extended periods of starvation were unintentional in the past, the thousands of years of repeating patterns of fasting, eating and fasting again, eventually became a norm and got embedded in our system. Since our genetic make-up adapted, it enabled our body to optimize its functions even during a fasted state. In fact, evidence shows that fasting has become an integral part of human's natural biochemical processes, wherein absence of prolonged fasts is thought to be the root cause of certain metabolic dysfunctions that people are suffering today. Simply put, perpetual eating is detrimental to our health.

EF's immediate effect is weight loss coming from mostly water and fat loss. And it is simply due to absence of nutrient intake that sets your body into fat-burning mode, as compared to fed state, as in eating, wherein your body is simply in the fat-storing mode.

If you've never really fasted long enough or engaged in energy-spending activities enough to activate lipolysis (fat-burning), your entire life is practically a pile up of fat-storing years, leading to an existence dominated by fat-building up mechanism. Both fat-burning and fat-storage phases of our bodily functions are set in motion without our active involvement and without clear notice from our conscious brain.

In the previous edition, I was quick to recommend a 7-day EF regime for those who want to jumpstart the process, know their capacity, and maximize weight loss within the shortest possible time. However, knowing what many know now, I've seen much greater and sustainable progress among those who became fat-adapted first without fasting, and that is through low carbohydrate, moderate to high fat & protein intake for at least two weeks before jumping in the fasting wagon. This way, there is a smooth transition in your system, so your cells slowly recognize fats and ketones as its major source of energy without sensing threat and hunger.

Now, if you are already fat-adapted and open to EF for whatever healthful reason you consider, you may continue learning more about it in the following texts.

With proper mindset and some extras to help you during EF, it is said that in general, a person has an average of six weeks fat allowance to sustain a clean fast. Some fasting gurus say that the real magic and wonder happen after the 21st day, when tumors reduce in size, mental clarity is activated at its optimum, and most medical conditions are reversed.

If it is hard for you to imagine, let's do a little math again (*not biochemically perfect, but a good estimate*):

- Six weeks is 42 days
- If a 70 kg man needs 2,000 kcal on a regular day, he will need 84,000 calories to survive those six weeks (2,000 kcal x 42 days = 84,000 kcal in 42 days)
- Since 1g of fats can yield 9 kcal, a person can just lose 9.3 kg of fats to provide that (84,000kcal / 9 kcal / 1g of fats= 9,333 grams of fats)
- This way, one can imagine that a 10-kg of extra fat weight, something many can spare, can already provide calories good for six weeks.

If one is coming from a previous lifestyle that piled up a lot of inflammation and visceral fats, without the delicate metabolic problems needing medications, a minimum of seven days fasting can be considered. On the other hand, if your schedule will not allow you as of this point, a 5-day extended fast is reasonable because you will have at least a day of reaching full ketosis and fat burning level that is good enough for you to be inspired to do it again.

(Reminder: DO NOT DO IT NOW. Finish this book first, learn other materials, if necessary, ask professional advice, and study yourself well.)

Below is a sample table of a seven-day fasting protocol with the corresponding preparations, expectations, and results.

Engaging in EF for more than seven days might require additional vitamin & mineral supplements as discussed in the previous chapters.

This is a simple approximation of when glycolysis, glycogenolysis, gluconeogenesis, and lipolysis/ketosis occur on average. Certain people will have variation depending on their glycogen and muscle stores.

Although I highly recommend a 5-7-day jumpstart EF after being fat-adapted, you can design it to fit your own lifestyle, either longer or shorter. It is said that when your hunger starts to recur, especially when there's no trigger like visual or smell stimulation, that is a good sign to break your fast, regardless of your fasting schedule.

Again, variations of *fat fasting* may be opted, but I personally do not recommend such especially before you know how you can really perform on a clean fast, like this sample schedule:

Day 1 and 2: Expect to be at your hungriest, take only minimal water and salt whenever you feel hungry, thirsty, or light-headed. Rest and lie down if necessary. For those who have been incorporating dry fasting in their daily routine like me, I feel that day 1-2 is easier if it's done on DF. Assess yourself as time goes by. It is also helpful to schedule things to do. I personally recommend a task that is cognitively stimulating, but physically less demanding.

Day 3 to 5: Hunger is more tolerable; you can add magnesium 1-2 tablets per day if with strenuous physical activity and symptoms and evidence of hypomagnesemia.

Day 6 to 7: Hunger may occasionally be more prominent, make sure you are well hydrated both with water and electrolytes. If you have muscle pains/cramps despite adequate sodium and magnesium, you can add potassium on this day. Once you decide to break your fast, it must be done the proper way and NEVER

ABRUPTLY to avoid side effects.

The question of when to do it is also as important. And for me, the answer is the soonest that you can. If you do not have important events where food intake is inevitable like a wedding in the family, birthday of someone special, or a golden wedding anniversary, then fasting can be done immediately. In fact, you can do it during your most routinary week and some even suggest doing it when you are expecting to be at your busiest. That way, your mind will be taken away from food and your body will easily shift to "hunting" mode, thereby increasing your focus and concentration. And before you know it, your day is already done.

Being a married woman now, it is an addition for me to check that I am not pregnant before I engage in an extended fast.

As I have previously mentioned, the challenge in fasting is basically 80-95% psychological and only 5-20% physical. That major challenge can easily be countered by equipping yourself with the knowledge that you are truly physiologically capable. Mentally prepare yourself for all the expected manifestations of fasting and embrace episodes of hunger knowing that such negative sensation is only staying for a fleeting moment. Once addressed, the minimal physical struggle can even be less.

To discuss more on the types of EF and their applicability in certain situations, here are the common variations:

ADF or Alternate Day Fasting

This is when you fast for a day, proceed with a regular eating time the following day, and fast the next, alternatively.

If you eat regularly at the same time, this will give you 36 hours of fasting and 12 hours eating window every two days.

This can be done when one already reaches a normal BMI but wants to lose pounds little by little to a more comfortable and lighter body without engaging in longer fasts.

24-Hour Fasting Protocol 2-3x a Week

This is when one engages in a 24-hour fasting two to three times per week. This protocol can be done during the maintenance phase for those who are always busy. This way, time can be maximized since food preparation is reduced to once every other day. Caloric and other nutrient needs should be obtained during feeding days to avoid undesirable excessive weight loss.

42-Hour Fasting Protocol

In this schedule, you have a 6-hour eating window every other day, providing a 42-hour fasting in between. This is usually done by those with very slow metabolism for them to jumpstart weight loss without engaging in longer fasts.

This is also perfect for those who have a very busy schedule who want to maximize their time without getting bothered by food intake every now and then.

Extended Fasting Greater than Three Days

This is usually done after a long-planned indulgence like holidays or vacations with intake of inflammatory foods, or to break a plateau or to jumpstart on ketosis every now and then. Once you are in this fasting lifestyle, EF will just be part of your toolbox and you will instinctively know when you will need to do it.

Note that during the first try, when you are not yet adapted to fasting, there will be signs of hypoglycemia that usually accompany your hunger pangs. This will include tremors, cold sweats, and some degree of lightheadedness. If this occurs, you can rest for a while or drink water with salt and observe. If this persists, you can add 99 mg potassium, low dose magnesium or take bone broth and see if it will improve. On the other hand, if your condition continues to worsen, immediately terminate the fast and slowly introduce food to your system. Note that for some, it may take several attempts to successfully complete a planned EF, and there is no shame in that. Each attempt will have a benefit of its own and the eventual success will be worth it.

Other uncomfortable, temporary but generally harmless, changes that may occur during EF are as follows:

- *Absent or reduced bowel movement*
- *Body odor or bad "acetone" breath from ketosis*
- *Headache during the early days*
- *Sleep disturbance or shortened sleep cycle*
- *Restlessness*
- *Food cravings*
- *Irritability with heightened emotions*

These "side effects" can easily be managed and seldom cause serious problems, especially that the benefits strongly outweigh those risks. However, if this is not enough to convince you to do an extended fast, then, don't. Extended fasting is not the exclusive way to lose weight. But it is the fastest and most natural way to do it. And I find it very useful in keeping the fat loss I already accomplished. Note that sustaining the weight loss will need the normalization of hunger and satiety hormones, which can be achieved by breaking the lifelong frequent eating routine so many of us are used to.

Multiple *EFs* may be done before one can reach their ideal weight. However, if after trying and EF is something that you cannot do outright, do not worry because there is still a way to lose those extras long-term.

For a slower yet smoother weight loss transition, intermittent fasting can be done instead.

CHAPTER 9

Intermittent Fasting

"Periodic fasting can help clear up the mind and strengthen the body and the spirit."

- Ezra Taft Benson

Simply known as IF, this new name to an old practice has different variations. If this is the first time that you have heard of it and is not certain that you can do it, you can make an assessment by mentally counting the hours from the time you usually have your dinner at night, and the time you have your breakfast in the morning. If it is less than 12 hours, then you can slowly extend it to 12, by either eating dinner early or moving your breakfast a little later the next day.

Remember that your bedtime milk or hot chocolate counts, so you can also start by skipping that or drinking caffeine-free tea instead.

Slowly, you can increase your fasting period by the hour each day, depending on your activities, schedule, goals, and preference.

Once you get the hang of it, you can proceed until you reach 16 hours fasting and an 8-hour eating window, where you can eat as normally as you would. That is called a 16:8 schedule which is a common variation. You can adjust your eating window based on your usual day. With a minimum of 16 hours fast and a maximum of eight hours of eating window, you can skip at least one major meal, like breakfast or dinner, or lump two meals into one like brunch.

At first, you may tend to overeat during your window, but overtime, you should learn that the time lost in fasting doesn't mean a time lost on eating that you should compensate after. Instead, think of it as a time well-spent allowing your body to burn fat, and those undesirable fats that luckily got burned, need not be replaced, especially immediately.

You will be surprised at how easy it is, especially when you are at your busiest in the morning, to skip breakfast and even lunch. After a month or so, you can lengthen it to 18:6 or even 20:4. It is important that you listen to your body when you eat. This is the practice of mindful eating. Don't eat simply because your window is open. Instead, eat slowly when you are hungry and stop the moment you feel satisfied. An 8-hour eating window does not mean an 8-hour of nonstop eating. Instead, you can plan two proper meals with or without a light snack in between.

As you move your fasting window longer, know that the benefits are also multiplying by the hour. The 19:5 is advocated by Dr.

Atkin in his book where he noted that by reducing one's eating window to five hours, you can skip two meals, making it a One Meal A Day routine or OMAD. This can also be done in 20:4 schedules. Some even do it as long as 22:2 but this has a risk of lowering your overall metabolism, thus, I personally do not recommend doing it daily, but can be incorporated a few days in a week. What is great about fasting is that it is very flexible, especially during special occasions or dinner out, where you can simply adjust on a day-to-day basis, so long as you do not go below what I consider the minimum 16 hours regular fasting. Initially, you may need to count your fasting hours starting from the last food intake of the previous day. Overtime, this will become a habit and you will no longer need to be conscious about time and you start to do it naturally.

Again, note that OMAD does not mean a single meal alone. You can open your window by having some light snacks, like a salad or a soup, an avocado or 2 poached eggs. After 30 minutes or an hour, you can proceed with your main meal with your choice of meat or whatever that you are happy with. And just before closing your window, you can drink some coffee if it is still early, and some Low Carb nuts and natural cheese if you still feel like it.

OMAD is known to break the *Ghrelin-Leptin* hormonal imbalance most people are suffering in this modern day. It is also one of the best ways to maintain your fat loss once you've reached your goal weight. This can be done without continuous weight loss and preservation of muscle mass when paired with high protein intake, weightlifting, and ample amount of sleep.

For beginners and those who have maximized fat loss, doing **Circadian Fasting** is the easiest and most sustainable way of starting your IF journey. This is done through daily fasting of at least 12 hours, with emphasis on one's last meal at 4-6 hours before bedtime, regardless of their sleeping time. This way, the body can truly rest and rejuvenate while asleep and not be consumed by the demands of digestion. Circadian Fasting is also best done by those with irregular work-sleep schedules, that usually disrupts an individual's metabolism. This pattern of eating harmonizes well with the body's evolutionary routine, thus, optimizes its function, including correction of hormonal imbalance, repair of damaged cellular parts, production of necessary proteins, and cleansing of our drainage (lymphatic) system.

Other benefits of *fasting* include appetite correction, regularization of bowel movement, economical savings, more time and focus on more important matters, and freedom from food dependence.

CHAPTER 10

Factors Affecting Fat Loss While Fasting

"The discipline of fasting breaks you out of the world's routine."

-Jentezen Franklin

If there is one word that you need to know in this weight loss journey, it should be that very thing that largely influences fasting and fat loss, and that is, insulin. Insulin is the hormone that is released whenever you take in food. It is essential but it should be kept at a lower level since fluctuations can easily lead to weight gain. The moment it is circulated in your bloodstream, your body sets off all the mechanisms of being in a *fed state,* and that would mean fat-storage. Insulin's other name is fat-storing hormone.

Insulin spike sends a signal to your brain that it is the time of abundance, like the harvest season, or a successful hunting trip, in human's early evolution. Thus, our body being remarkably amazing and frugal as it is, will save all the extra food you eat and store it in the form of glycogen and fats for future fasting use.

Generally, all calorie-containing foods and to some extent, zero calorie sweeteners, trigger insulin secretion, but in hierarchy, carbohydrates (especially refined carbohydrates in large doses) is the most potent stimulus, followed by proteins and the least stimulating of all, fats. Thus, consumption of any of those can break your fast and eventually jeopardize the fat loss in fasting by halting fat-burning. It is the reason why avoidance of food must be done at all costs during fasting, in order for you to see the results you are trying to achieve.

Note that you can eat again during your window, but fat loss is maximized and may be continued if you consume healthy and natural protein and fat-rich food (instead of carbohydrates) while not fasting.

It is at this point that we will discuss the basic truths about the food we consume, so that we can better understand and maneuver our ways both during fasting and feasting periods.

Food can be divided into three macronutrients, namely Carbohydrates, Proteins, and Fats. These are the generalities of the three:

Carbohydrates include bread, rice, pasta, potatoes, cereals, cakes, pastries, and most fruits. They are known to give us energy and back in our elementary school days, they were the ones that can be seen in the **Go** part of *Go, Grow and Glow Food Chart*.

Chemistry-wise, its basic unit is **Glucose**. In layman's term, this simply equates to **sugar,** *although technically, sugar is a mixture of both glucose and fructose.* Remember, excess carbohydrates are stored as glycogen, and glycogen has very limited storage space largely in the liver. Consuming extra carbohydrates after your glycogen capacity is full leads to its conversion into fats.

Physiologically speaking, there is no such thing as essential carbohydrate, simply because we can create it *de novo* or from scratch. Thus, we can live without consuming any of it. Unfortunately, we generally consume more of this least essential macronutrient that superlatively leads to insulin spike, thus making this the top offender in jeopardizing fat loss.

Proteins on the other hand, commonly come from meaty, fishy, and beefy food sources. This would include all lean meat of fish, pork, beef, chicken, white part of eggs, mushrooms and most parts of beans and nuts. Its basic component is **Amino Acid.** This equates to *Grow* in the food pyramid. Some glucogenic amino acid can be converted to glucose, and if consumed in excess, can also lead to fat stores. Most amino acids are recyclable and can be made by our own cells. However, there are essential amino acids that need to be consumed from food since we do not have the enzymes or equipment in our cells to produce them *de novo*. To some extent, proteins also increase insulin release, though its elevation is just modest. So long as you consume proteins together with at least a moderate amount of fats and minimal carbohydrates, fat storage will not be at a detrimental level.

Once you reach adulthood, our need for proteins is less as compared to growing children. With usual physical activity, we require an average of 1 gram of protein per kilogram of body weight to avoid muscle wasting.

Simply put, if you are a 70 kg man, with an average lifestyle, you can consume approximately 70 grams of protein in a day to avoid muscle loss. As per serving sizes, one matchbox of meat is 28 grams, that contains about seven grams of proteins. Thus, a total of 10 matchbox sizes of meat is needed as per minimum.

However, this protein need is quite low if we are going to avoid the insulin-spiking carbohydrates. Regular meal usually comprises 50-70% Carbohydrates, 30-40% Proteins, and 10% Fats. Thus, in a Low Carb way of eating that promotes continued fat loss, proteins can be eaten at about 2-3 grams per kilogram of body weight, with moderate fat intake of one to one and a half grams of fats per body weight. The total calories would then be a little less than a full number needed for maintenance of that weight.

Too much protein without fats in meals can still lead to weight gain due to absence of ketosis via increased insulin release.

This metabolic equivalent usually comes as a huge surprise for many. But this is also the reason why those who are on a high-protein diet, without engaging in enough strenuous physical activity, are continuously gaining extra weight in the form of fats or hidden visceral fats, overtime. Thus, to maintain low insulin levels, protein consumption should also be regulated.

Lastly, **Fats**. These are complex molecules that are generally oily, also known as lipids. Among the three macros, fats are the most underrated, confused, and wrongly accused. Popularly known to cause heart problems and complications, fats are what can sustain life during prolonged fasting in the form of fatty acids and **ketones** as a fuel source. Note that fats are not converted to glucose or proteins, and pure natural fats are not an efficient stimulus for insulin secretion, making this the most fat-loss friendly macro. Triglycerides, a special kind of lipid in the body, can forego its glycerol backbone to be made into glucose for certain cells in the body that will need it, like Red Blood Cells.

Common forms of fats include lard or pork fats, tallow or beef fats, cooking oil, butter, egg yolk, fats from animal products, and full cream dairies. It is also the basic fuel source for our heart in the form of triglycerides and fatty acids. And yes, it is the basic fact as to why we are informed that we must do our cardio exercises if we want to lose the fats that are circulating in our bloodstream.

Not known to all, fats are part of the *Go* in our food chart. It becomes an energy fuel in the form of fatty acid and ketones once metabolized, and a very efficient energy source, not just for the heart but also for the brain and majority of the processes in our body. Like proteins, there is also what we call *essential fats*. These are the kind of fats that must be taken externally for our body to function properly. If consumed exclusively in our diet, or in high quantity in proportion to small part of proteins and carbohydrates, insulin spike becomes less likely, which also means that fat-storing mechanism is also on hold and weight gain now is at minimum, if none at all, especially at an amount not surpassing one's daily basic caloric needs.

Fat intake only becomes a problem if it is consumed together with ample amounts of carbohydrates and proteins. This meal ratio will facilitate energy consumption from the easily dispensable glucose and proteins, which leads to increased insulin secretions. This increased insulin secretion will not burn the fats as energy but store it in your body in many forms. It can be stored in your liver (thus causing fatty liver), as peripheral or what we call as subcutaneous fats (like in your thighs and arms), visceral fats (the one dangerously covering your internal organs, intestines, heart, etc.) or worse, as a bad cholesterol circulating your bloodstream.

The latter form of fats are the free fats in our vascular system known as LDL (Low Density Lipoprotein), but the worst kind is VLDL (Very Low-Density Lipoprotein) and other remnant cholesterol. High LDL in the absence of inflammatory markers are shown to be not as dangerous in the current studies. But high

LDL with high insulin, high blood sugar and elevated markers of inflammation like ESR and CRP are considered high risk for cardiovascular events and are the ones causing problems like hypertension, heart attack, and stroke. However, if fat intake is not paired with insulin-spiking foods, then, the fats you consume will be utilized as energy and will not be stored the way it could have been if insulin is also high.

Another important aspect that we need to recognize is the fact that refined carbohydrates do not trigger the satiety center in our brain. Meaning, it will not make you feel full or satisfied or that you've had enough. Instead, you keep on eating and eating until you feel that you are about to throw up or your stomach about to burst. You feel full but that sense of fullness is not the same sense of fullness you get by eating an avocado with slices of bacon and egg. It is because the satiety center in the brain is activated by proteins and fats, and not by pure carbohydrates.

Thus, if you are keen enough, you will notice that following a full meal, you can no longer take another tenderloin steak, but you can still accommodate a slice of cake. The carbohydrates from cake will not communicate your fullness to your brain, hence, it is negated as far as your fullness signal is concerned. Thus, this is another reason why carbohydrate intake, especially in the form of simple sugar, must be taken with utmost care. Your brain may not recognize it, but you yourself should take heed and do what is needed.

Glow foods on the other hand can be found incorporated within those three macronutrients. These are micronutrients we need in minuscule amounts for all the biochemical processes in our body to go smoothly. Generally, these are the vitamins and minerals known as A to Z. Thus, if there is a kind of food you want to eat, you make sure it has less sugar and is loaded with these nutrients since overtime, especially after fasting, these micronutrients should be replenished.

CHAPTER 11

When and How to Break a Fast

"Fasting is the first principle of medicine. Fast and see the strength of the spirit reveal itself."

-Rumi

Engaging in fasting, especially extended ones, puts your gastrointestinal system in a temporary phase of relaxation. While the rest of your body might be active from the influx of energy from ketones, your gut is simply enjoying the calm that absence of food intake brings.

The moment you are adapted to fasting, your body simply goes on getting used to ketones as fuel source. By essence, the only essential parts of our body that are made of fats are our brain and nerves, which is only about 2% of our overall body composition in males and about 10% in females (which have more necessary fats for reproductive purposes). Thus, theoretically speaking in general, as long as our body fat percentage does not go down below 5% in men and 12% in women, we can continue to live on a fasted state while consuming only electrolytes and other essential vitamins and minerals, as did the research volunteer, Angus Barbieri, who fasted for the all-time record of 382 days and lost about 200 kg after.

Yet, realistically speaking, it is not just practical to fast all at once until you lose all the excess fats and reach your ideal weight. During this journey, there will be a lot of times when you will be breaking your fast and it is important to know when and how to properly do so.

By experience, when to break a fast is largely a case-to-case basis.

Some fasting experts say that the return of hunger after days of loss of appetite serves as a good signal to break a fast. But personally, I consider this very subjective. Knowing that appetite can be stimulated by mere sight or smell of food, return of hunger may just be a physiologic manifestation of a psychological response to external factors, like an advertisement of a fast-food chain or the scent of your favorite meal or the sight of your lunch buddy.

If you want to be very objective about it, you can monitor your body fat percentage daily while following an EF protocol. There are several methods for estimating body fat percentage, including:

1. Skinfold measurements: This involves using calipers to pinch and measure the thickness of skin and subcutaneous fat at various points on the body.

2. Bioelectric impedance analysis (BIA): This method uses a

small electrical current to estimate body fat by measuring the resistance of body tissues to the current.

3. Dual-energy X-ray absorptiometry (DXA): This is a medical imaging technique that uses X-rays to measure bone density, lean mass, and fat mass.

4. Hydrostatic weighing: This method involves weighing a person underwater to calculate their body density, which can then be used to estimate body fat.

5. Air displacement plethysmography (ADP): Also known as the Bod Pod, this method measures body composition using air displacement to calculate body volume.

It's important to note that no method is 100% accurate, but these methods can help provide a general estimate of body fat percentage.

As a rule, you lose about half pound of pure body fats per 24 hours of fasting. And if you are doing generally well with fasting, and is not nearing the critical body fat percentage, you can continue to do so as you wish. You can then intentionally break your fast when you finally reach your goal, whether that is a goal weight, body image, percent body fat, or even goal activities (that includes things you always wanted to do but cannot do so because of the extra pounds). But other than that, a good enough reason for me to break a fast is being contented with the progress I have made so far, being fulfilled with the accomplishment of completing a planned fast, or a task I wanted to finish while fasting, and a conscious decision to go back to the dining table and enjoy the food in the company of people that I love spending time and celebrating life with. And once I decide when I will break my fast, the next thing I do is plan on how I will do it.

In fasting and in most life's undertakings, it is true what the song advocates, *"if you have to break it, break it gently"*.

In general, the longer you fast, the gentler you should be in re-introducing food into your system.

After your last intended day of fasting, you can slowly consume light calorie-containing food like a vegetable soup or bone broth.

Since your insulin level at this point is at an all-time low, your body has become more sensitive to anything that can increase it, thus it is best to avoid simple, processed/refined sugars. Foods with very strong flavors or with dense composition, like lean meat, are better reserved for the third to fourth meal after fasting as this can cause indigestion since your gut has been inactive for so long and should not be forced to function fully all at once.

There are many ways to break a fast. By thoroughly planning your fasting days until you break it, you will have a smoother transition during your period of "re- feeding" and you will have less chances of having a *"re-feeding syndrome"*, wherein abrupt ending of an extended fast followed by a very heavy meal results to a medical emergency that comes from sudden changes of metabolites and electrolytes in a previously nutrient-deprived individual. The chances of this incidence from occurring is very low, especially when you follow clean fasting with basic electrolyte supplementation and is not extending this for months, but it is still a risk I do not approve for anyone to be taking.

Personally, after a 7-day fast, I recommend breaking it with one bowl of soup at the first hour and followed by a light meal one to two hours after. Close your window after another two hours with another light meal.

The following day, you can proceed with your preferred maintenance IF schedule, but with lighter meals than usual and continue to do so until the third to fourth day when a regular full meal can now be consumed.

As a rule, for longer Dry Fasting, the *"breakfast protocol"* should last as long as the days of DF before resumption of regular diet. For example, a three-day DF should have three days of protocol, like simple fluids with electrolytes on day 1, bone broth and soup on day 2, and light proteins like eggs and softened meat on day 3.

Whereas for regular Wet Fasting, the minimum breakfast protocol can be shortened to have the time of fasting. For example, three days of WF can have a full day of light soup and half a day of light proteins, before proceeding to a full low carb, non-insulin spiking, and without refined carbs kind of meal. Certain foods are also advised as part of breakfast protocol but may not be essential for others who are already adapted.

1. Bone broth with electrolytes
2. Light vegetables
3. Probiotics like kimchi, plain yogurt, sauerkraut, or kombucha
4. Light proteins like eggs and fish

As much as possible, avoid breaking your fast with sugar, other refined carbohydrates, and those loaded with white grains or breads, as this can lead to insulin spike, hyperstimulation syndrome, and eventual syncope from sudden peak and dip of blood glucose level. Reread this chapter as needed until a good and basic breakfast protocol is known by heart. For daily short IF, however, only a few needs slower reintroduction of food. If you do not have a sensitive gut, you may just proceed with your normal breakfast instead.

CHAPTER 12

Foods that Enhance Fat Loss

"The philosophy of fasting calls upon us to know ourselves, to master ourselves, and to discipline ourselves the better to free ourselves."
-Tariq Ramadan

As what we previously discussed, carbohydrates, and to some extent, too much proteins with little to zero fats, are the main cause of spikes in insulin, which eventually leads to fat storing mechanism and eventually weight gain.

Unfortunately, the danger of overconsumption of those macros doesn't stop there. Continuous influx of carbs leads to fat cells becoming *insulin* and *leptin- resistant*. With that kind of hormonal resistance, your body won't be able to know when you have had enough. It is a vicious cycle where you keep on eating all those foods, storing them as fats, yet no signal comes to your brain that you are already full and satisfied. As a result, complications of elevated blood sugar occur. Fats that can no longer be deposited on your arms and legs are now circulating your bloodstream. That bad cholesterol, together with inflammation which freely circulates your system, will eventually clog your arteries, leading to high blood pressure, heart attack, or stroke.

Thus, if you want to maintain fat loss during your eating window, you must seriously consider a low carbohydrate, moderate to high proteins, and moderate to high fat diet.

Out of hundreds of diet fads out there that may seem to be contradicting with each other, a common theme of foods is actually binding all of them.

In general:

Eat whole foods.
Eat only the edible foods you know were picked or harvested from plants that grew from soil or meat that previously walked or flew or swam. The more you eat them in their natural (and sanitary) state, the better. Yes, all raw edibles you can think of that can be made into a salad is included.

Eat less processed foods.
As a rule, avoid everything that comes in packaging except for pure coconut oil for cooking, virgin olive oil consumed uncooked, real butter, full fat dairy products, and real egg-yolk mayonnaise if you cannot make it yourself (*yes, you can come up with a 1-2-minute do-it-yourself-mayonnaise*).

At least 80% of the time, I try to stick to a single-step food processing rule, that is, I will eat only those that were processed once, like a grilled pork belly or fried chicken. Sparingly, I accommodate two-step processed foods like (1) fried (2) smoked bacon. And because I am a mere fallible mortal, I allow for three- or more-step processed foods on special days but not exceeding 20% of my consumption (i.e. Low Carb Cake, Pastry or other desserts).

No simple sugar on a regular basis.

Avoid as much as you can all types of table sugar, bread, pastries, cakes, potatoes especially ready-to- cock mashed ones, sodas and flavored drinks, beer, and flavored alcoholic drinks.

Think of portions when you eat.

Not just in quantity but also in quality. In general, you can fill up one large plate with high fiber, low carbohydrate veggies, and another smaller plate with some proteins like eggs and something sumptuous like pork steak. Isn't that mouth-watering?

See below the list on the food you can eat that can still help weight loss even when eaten until satisfaction. The suggested ratio of a maximum of 20 grams carbohydrates (see options below), 2-3 grams of protein/kg of body weight of protein and 1-1.5-gram fats/kg of body weight per day. (*See appendix* B)

Note that by eating a low carbohydrate, low to moderate proteins, and high fat diet, or *a Ketogenic Diet*, it will biochemically mimic ketosis, thus will put you in a state like that when one is engaging in prolonged fasting despite only doing IF. This is just reserved for those who cannot do a clean fast.

Approved Green List of Foods You Can Eat Freely

Carbohydrates – must contain 0-5 grams of net carbohydrates per 100 grams, eaten fresh, cooked or fermented like kimchi or pickled, as long as there is no added sugar.

- All green leafy vegetables like spinach, cabbage, brussel sprouts, malunggay, lettuce, sweet potato leaves, kangkong and many more.

- Low-carbohydrate vegetables – cauliflower, broccoli, bell peppers, asparagus, cucumber, zucchini, celery, radishes

- Fruits – generally, all fruits are high in carbohydrate content; small portions of berries, avocado and mature coconut meat may be eaten when a "dessert" is necessary.

Proteins – proteins should be prioritized as this is shown to improve metabolism, prevent excessive weight loss, and correct appetite. Generally, about 100 grams of protein can be obtained from half a kilo of lean, raw meat, and is a safe estimate for those in the 50 to 70-kg weight range.

- All animal meat and meat products cured in natural

processes, including sausages and salami, eggs, offal/internal organs and seafood, are great sources of quality proteins. Few exceptions are fishes known to have high mercury content like swordfish, tilefish, among others.

- Plant-based proteins – most nuts in limited amounts (almonds, peanuts, flaxseed, chia, macadamia, pecan, pumpkin seeds, sunflower seeds, walnuts), mushrooms, and certain organic beans.

Fats – healthy, natural fats should be the primary source of energy or daily caloric requirements. Although you can generally eat all that you want, make sure that you only eat when you are hungry and stop eating as soon as you are full or satisfied. Avoid eating sweet foods to counter the feelings of being "fed up". Instead, listen to your body and just stop eating because it's a good signal that you've really had enough. Although you would still be in ketosis if you eat more than what you will need, however, your body will burn the energy coming from the fats you consume and not the extra fats stored in your body. That is why, when one still has a lot of fats that need burning, control of fat intake is also beneficial. Here is a list of healthy fats you can take during your window:

- *Plant-based* – Avocado oil, coconut milk and oil, olives and olive oil, certain nuts (walnut) and seeds (flaxseed, chia seeds).

- *Animal-based* – All full-cream dairy products, natural

cheeses, yogurt, egg yolk, homemade cream, cream cheese, all types of animal fat from beef, pork, chicken, duck or salmon, butter, ghee, duck fat, and full-fat mayonnaise.

Other food products:

Any condiments and seasonings without added sugar, preservatives, and vegetable oil, like pepper, cinnamon, cayenne powder, dried herbs, natural spices and many more can be used.

Sweeteners – ideally should be avoided as this still cause insulin spike despite low sugar content, but when necessary, opt for the following: erythritol granules in 15 g or less in a day, stevia leaves/powders, xylitol granules, allulose, and monk fruit.

Know more about these in our food list in Appendix F.

CHAPTER 13

Foods to Avoid in Fat Loss

"Start the practice of self-control with penance; begin with fasting."

-Mahavira

As you can see, the worst type of food when in the process of fat loss are carbohydrates, especially sugar.

However, you might think that taking away carbs, also means taking away your joy.

Don't be overdramatic; you know that is not true. With the internet and thousands of food geniuses sharing their knowledge, you can practically have almost everything in low carbohydrate, real sugar-free alternative. Don't believe me? Try Googling "Low Carb Dinner Rolls Recipe" and you won't miss out on the real thing.

You see, I believe the favorite kinds of carbs can be divided into three types: first are those that neutralize a sumptuous main course, like a mashed potato or a simple pasta, rice, or bread. Secondly, there are carbohydrates that are needed because they provide bulk that most individuals are used to having in their bowel movement. And lastly, it makes up most of our desserts. And since we cannot completely do away with it, it is important that we try to understand carbohydrates better so we can manage our intake sparingly, yet still be successful with our journey to better health.

First, let's tackle why we are so used to having something bland or less tasteful to accompany a perfectly good steak? This can be understood by examining the following major reasons:

Economical - It may no longer be applicable to you now, but as expenses are part of day-to-day life, two cups of mashed potato is still cheaper than another slice of steak. Thus, with less cost, you will be "filled" faster. So, if you are not saving, you can do away with it. And if like me, you are also conscious with your spending, there are so many low carbohydrate alternatives that are affordable to pair with your favorite steak or eat more affordable meats like regular beef, pork, chicken, and fish.

Too much flavor makes you feel fed-up easily - When you are eating something very delicious, like a slab of roast pork, no matter how much you like it, you can only consume a certain amount and you know you can no longer take another bite after. Unless you accompany it with something with lesser flavor, to "neutralize" it. Although it is truly understandable, you must recognize that the feeling of "fullness", satisfied, and satiated even if you've just eaten less than half of what your stomach can accommodate, is a normal bodily function that we should be very sensitive about. Again, it is the fats and proteins that trigger that Satiety Center in our brain and not the carbohydrates. So, if you are feeling "satiated", you can just stop eating and drink coffee, tea, or water to fill up the remaining space. However, if like me, you also want the physical feeling of fullness, then I recommend you take note of the alternatives on the green list that you can eat as much as you can, without worrying about the carbohydrate count.

It is essential in our daily and bulky toilet routines – Yes, many need carbohydrates to do their favorite morning alone time, but this is only by habit not a real requirement for good health. Some experts suggest that daily bowel movement is more of a psychological routine rather than a physical need. A lot of us feel good after some bowel elimination, thus, the incorporation of some amount of carbohydrates is mostly preferred. But remember that what you need is a specific kind of carbohydrate called dietary fiber. These fibers will give bulk to your stool to eliminate wastes properly. With adequate water intake, your toilet moments will still go smoothly so long as you consume a low carbohydrate, high fiber meal. It is also important to note that fiber is also a major contributor in constipation. That is why there are individuals like me who are sensitive to fibers and have better bowel movement when avoiding it. Just know that when one is eating a low-residue, low-fiber meal like a carnivore, it is expected to have a stool that is smaller in quantity as compared to the opposite. (*See the vegetable options in the green list if you wish to have larger stool bulk.*)

Lastly, who can live without desserts? Surely, many can't. Although I have tried especially during the first few months, I completely eradicated all the sweets I've known my whole life. I decided to enroll myself in a self-imposed *"Sugar Addiction Rehabilitation"*, and I believe I succeeded for two straight months. After, I then slowly reintroduced sweets in our kitchen with the good kind. And this time, with control. I make large batches of low-carb fat bombs and chocolate puddings and amazingly almost never touch them in my fridge. I tricked my brain with the idea that I have an ample supply of sweets that I can go to anytime, and with that, my interest just died down. As a rule, I do not use simple sugars. As an alternative, I use Stevia or *Monkfruit* sweetener; these are natural, organic, low to zero calorie sweeteners you can use with caution. And since they cost more than table sugar and still stimulate the same pleasure center in our brain and to some extent, elevate insulin despite being zero-calorie content, I use them at minimum and the final dessert, I eat only when I have cravings that now occur very rarely.

For further guidance, see the Unapproved Red List below on foods that can jeopardize your journey towards ideal body weight. In general, these are processed foods, sugary, artificial, some whole but carbo-loaded foods like pasta, rice, noodles, potatoes, cereals and even most fruits. Also, for best outcome, kindly avoid cigarette smoking and alcohol consumption, in addition to food that you eat during an open window, until our two months of clean eating target is reached.

Note that when one is still in the process of losing weight, EF is recommended. But if only IF is feasible, then it is strongly suggested to do it with the right foods and avoid all that's in the danger list as possible.

This way, you will be able to see results as if you are engaging in EF as well.

Unapproved Red List Foods to be Avoided

In general, these food options are not essential for your survival. It may activate the pleasure center in your brain (*the same center triggered by illicit drugs like cocaine*) and subsequently, sugar addiction, but it will do nothing good in your journey towards reaching your health goal. These may be eaten in very rare and special occasions and in portions, but never a weekly or even monthly routine.

- Traditional baked products – any food products containing flours, corn, wheat, rice, cassava, potato, or other starchy foods. These include bread, cookies, and pastries.

- All artificial drinks and fruits juices as these contain mostly either corn syrup, high amounts of fructose or artificial sweeteners.

- Processed dairy products, cheese spreads, coffee creamers, condensed milk, ice creams, rice and soy milk, and anything fat-free or low-fat counterpart.

- Toxic, processed fats like regular low-quality chocolates, seed oils, sunflower, vegetable and canola oils, vegetable oil-rich chocolate bars, syrups and related products, commercial sauces, margarines, and most prepared salad dressings.

- Fruits and vegetables – most fruits and vegetables not mentioned above are either high in sugar or fructose, refined carbohydrates of high calorie from starch like peas, potatoes, cassava, and excessive amounts of peanuts and legumes.

- Meat- unfermented soy or vegetarian proteins or vegemeat, meats cured mostly in sugar and other highly processed meat products like canned meats, sausages, and meat loafs.

- Sweeteners – all forms of sugar in various names like table sugar, brown, white, muscovado, coco sugar, artificial sweeteners, dried fruits, fructose, honey, candies, syrups and commercially prepared flavorings of any kind.

- General – all fast foods, junk foods, processed foods,

ultra-processed foods, instant food mixes because they usually use vegetable oils for frying, preservatives, processed poor quality meats and high carbohydrate products, and any food with added sugar.

Study this by heart in our food list in Appendix E.

CHAPTER 14

No Cheating, Make Plans Instead

"Fasting is necessary as feasting."

-Laila Gifty Akita

Celebrations are part of any social culture. And this lifestyle doesn't prohibit you from enjoying and indulging whenever the situation calls for it.

Single day celebrations like birthdays, weddings, and anniversaries don't need much adjustment. You can simply extend your fast the day before or after to fit the schedule. Note though that *Sunday Family Day*, as it occurs weekly, is no more special than Mondays or Wednesdays. Should you decide to indulge weekly, you might as well consider doing an extended fast each day after as well, just enough to burn all the extra calories you've taken. That's the beauty of this lifestyle; you can design it in your own personal way, with the knowledge in mind of how our body works and what fuel it burns, depending on how long you have fasted and what you've been consuming prior to fasting. This way, it's almost like it never happened.

The challenge usually comes during longer celebratory days like Christmas Season until New Year, or a long Thanksgiving week, or the vacation cruise you have been planning for years. The dictum on this would be the following:

- Enjoy the best way you can while considering food as a minor source of happiness. If unable to do so, consider below.

- Try doing at least 12-16 hours fasting. Breakfast buffets usually last until 10:00 in the morning, while dinner can start as early as 5PM, and you can end it by 6PM.

- Try sticking to low carbohydrate food choices, or at least have whole foods, if avoidance already jeopardizes your happiness.

- If all else fails, just enjoy the whole length and know when to get back to your routine as soon as your vacation is over. Since this is a lifestyle, you must go back to your normal, that is a combination of Low Carb with Fasting or LCF-kind of eating pattern. Sure, you would gain some pounds, but you will take it off in no time.

For you to avoid the feeling of guilt, plan your days ahead. Avoid using the term *cheat day* as this connotes dishonesty, something that is opposite to what we are aiming here. Instead, do some *planned indulgences*, where you will give in to foods and timing that is out of your routine for something special. This way, you will be able to have a harmonious relationship with food and you make sure you enjoy every bite and moments you share it with.

CHAPTER 15

What About Exercise

"The goal of fasting is inner unity."

-Thomas Merton

By now, you probably have the idea why exercise is not essential for weight loss. While it is true that the more energy you spend on exercising means the more calories you burn, the net effect may not necessarily be weight loss. As you know, a lot of factors are in place.

During an exercise routine, your body will consume energy like that when you are fasting. However, as you exercise, your metabolic rate or the amount of energy needed for you to function also increases.

This phenomenon, paired with depletion of electrolytes and muscle fatigue, will lead to increased demand for food. Hunger hormone *Ghrelin* will soar up high. Failure to deny what your body is craving will only lead to a rebound effect of consuming more than what you just probably need. And of course, we all know where that road leads.

In addition, studies show that extreme and strenuous exercises don't equate to sustained increase in metabolism, simply because our body adapts to it and our metabolism plateaus despite increased physical activity. Thus, it is another factor why it does not follow that the more you exercise, the more you lose weight, as seen in the famous television show, *The Biggest Loser*, or anybody you know who lost weight initially after going to the gym but gained it back or plateaued eventually.

But with the proper mindset and just the right amount of time and moderate intensity, exercise can boost weight loss in terms of fat stores. Wonder why I mentioned fat stores? It is because exercise can increase muscle bulk, and muscle weighs heavier than fats! That is why weight is actually not the best gauge for good health. In fact, we now recommend weight lifting and other resistance training in order to gain weight through mass, especially for those who have been very successful with low carb and fasting but were not able to preserve their lean body mass.

But if we are honest enough with ourselves, you know for sure whether what you have are muscles buried under the fats, or just fats above a thin muscle.

In addition, studies show that the more you exercise, it does not really lead to more fat loss from increased metabolism. This is because our body adapts to it, a.k.a. *metabolic adaptation,* thus making it less and less efficient as you increase your physical activities, unless you continue to augment your physical load each time. But know that it will only be up to a certain point, and haphazardly doing so can also take its toll when it comes to your heart and joints.

Don't get me wrong; I am not saying that you should not exercise because we know that exercise has numerous advantages like brain plasticity, endurance, improved sense of well-being, body contouring, physical strength, better immunity, stress endurance, cardiovascular health, and even some degree of anti-aging effects. These benefits can be attained just by having moderate exercise activity like running for 30 minutes 2 to 3 times a week, and alternately done with 5-10 minutes of High Intensity Interval Training or Weightlifting. But when it comes to weight loss alone, exercise is simply not required especially if you don't want to.

For those who are starting this way of life just now, exercise is recommended once you are already fat-adapted. That is, when one's body is already used to using fats as energy during fasting and even during eating windows as well.

For cardio exercises, you may strive to achieve a heart rate that is 180 minus your age, to avoid anaerobic metabolism. Ease in slowly and use exercise not as punishment but as a celebration of what your body can do.

CHAPTER 16

Weight Loss Plateau

"Fasting is not just a spiritual discipline; it can be a spiritual feast."

-Jentezen Franklin

When this occurs, ask yourself first if you really need to lose more weight or if you are already at your optimum for your height and age?

How long have you been in this lifestyle? Have you been following a clean low carb way of eating? Are you religious in sticking to your fasting schedule? Be honest with yourself and re-assess how you can improve your routine by starting again. Do not hurry and trust the process. Give it at least two full months before you jump into negative conclusions. There may be different factors to consider, and one possibility is because there are some who started with disrupted metabolism from a previous low calorie and other extreme diets, and may even experience weight gain during the first few weeks when the body was still adjusting.

Always remember that this lifestyle is not about perfection but continuous improvement. The progress that you make in making better choices each day and the commitment to get back on track as soon as you realize you unintentionally fell off the wagon is always an achievement in itself.

You sticking to this lifestyle even after achieving your goal signifies *self-love*. However, despite doing everything right and your weight loss plateaus, you may consider the following options:

Level up your fasting schedule. If you've been doing IF or 24H fasting, you can increase it one level higher (like from 14:10 to 16:8, or OMAD) or try doing a minimum of 36-48 hours of three days of extended fast. If you are not yet in your ideal goal, know that there is no plateauing in extended fasting especially when done right. Just make sure you are not underweight and you still have fats to lose (estimated to be more than 30% for females and more than 20% for males.)

Note that body fat percentage does not go below 10-12% which is considered the minimum with a safety net before you jeopardize neurological processes in your body. For young adult females, there might be a cap as to how much your body will allow you to lose, because this is a part of the evolutionary preservation of our most important function: to reproduce. Note that this body fat level is mostly seen in the subcutaneous layer and not the dangerous visceral fat nor the blood lipids. And as disappointing as it is for others, it is far from the body fat composition that commercial models have.

Try doing a *fat fast* for five days. This schedule is advocated by Dr. Atkin. In this protocol, you fast for five days, but each day, you can have five small all-fat intakes in a 5-hour eating period. Examples of fats you can consume are cream cheese with cocoa or nut butter, full fat heavy cream, MCT oil, grass-fed butter, full fat mayonnaise, and coconut cream. This protocol allows the individual to consume no more than 250 kcal of fat each time.

Check and recheck your meals, because even if you are doing LCF, you might have overlooked your protein & fat consumption. Excessive proteins can hinder fat loss and excessive calories from fats stops your body from burning your own fats. The muscle breakdown that happens during exercise is just minimal and the necessary proteins for repair and bulk formation can be obtained from the process of *autophagy*.

Do some measurements. For all you know, your body is reshaping. With *autophagy* that occurs especially when you are engaging in 24-hour fast or more, the fats are reduced, and the muscles improve in the right places.

And since muscles weigh more than fats, you might be really losing fats and gaining muscles. This is the reason why I advocate doing measurements like your arms, waist, hips, and neck circumference before starting anything. A mirror selfie on front, side, and back also provides a very good gauge and oftentimes better than the scale.

Check with your physician if you have other hormonal imbalance that could possibly lead to weight gain like *hypothyroidism* or *hyperaldosteronism* or *hyperinsulinemia*. Although these conditions can benefit from this lifestyle, certain conditions might need proper investigation and assistance from medications in order for it to be properly managed medically.

Check your prescriptions and ask your doctor if weight gain is a part of the side effects. If so, you can try asking if you can be slowly weaned from it (since fasting helps your body heal naturally) or find an alternative.

Double check your food portions. Although fasting boosts metabolism, after significant weight loss and especially drastic ones, your metabolism sometimes slows down. For others who started with slower metabolism, you might initially need to cut back a part of what you are consuming and follow an OMAD lifestyle for at least two months. After which, slowly increase your eating window to accommodate at least two meals a day. With this, your metabolism will normalize and as you become sensitive with your body, you will only eat when you really need to and stop when you are satisfied.

With these in mind, you can always have a back-up plan whenever you hit a bump along the way. Trust that it is possible. Trust that it is a proven science. Trust that you can do it and remember how much you want it in the first place. Always bear in mind your deep why.

CHAPTER 17

Why & How I Started Fasting

"Fasting is futile unless it is accompanied by an incessant longing for self-restraint."

-Mahatma Gandhi

Growing up, I have always felt that the way I look is not who I am inside. Despite reassurance from other people that I look and weighed "okay", a part of me always knew that I could do better, that I can be better. And it is only later that I realized that the physical improvement was just secondary, but how I healed myself psychologically, through discipline, self-control, and fasting, made all the difference.

I had asthma as a child and was diagnosed with allergic *rhinitis with conjunctivitis* during the later years. All my unfiltered pictures always show my *allergic shiners*, these are the dark circles around the eyes typical of people suffering from chronic inflammation and allergies. I have been maintaining an intranasal steroid and oral antihistamines for my allergies.

[You know I once kidded my friend that I am allergic to everything. And she said that it is impossible or else I'd be dead. I told her I am allergic to eye make-up and dogs, and that's practically everything. But seriously, my allergies already affected my everyday life.]

Because of my height and probably "sporty" build, I was always recruited for different games like basketball, soccer, lawn tennis, badminton, volleyball and even table tennis, and I engaged whenever the opportunity arose. But off intramural season, I would rather choose to be still: eat, sleep and enjoy the afternoon napping or chilling with my loved ones. As a result, I never really developed any muscles. And soon, I realized I have water retention, where my lower body becomes edematous later during the day. As a doctor, I know I only need to exercise to strengthen the muscles on my lower legs and improve my overall circulation. But I always find a good excuse not to exercise. One of my favorite excuses would be the idea that I am trying to live a minimalistic life, thus, doing physical exertion without actual work accomplishment, in the form of exercise, just doesn't seem to fit. Plus, I feel much better after a nap, more than anything.

Other than that, I feel like I am where I am meant to be; from career, relationship, personal development, and family. Food is the only aspect of my life that I am not in control with. Thus, I have decided that if I can gain control over food, I can gain control with any other aspects of my life.

This strong relationship with food runs in the family, especially on my paternal side. As sad as it is, he died only at the age of 56 due to complications of diabetes despite being very religious to his oral medications and insulin injection. He is only one among eight siblings, where four of them died one year apart, four years in a row due to various complications of diabetes, hypertension and subsequent kidney and heart disease.

Concerned that I may end up the same, I then began researching until I learned about fasting and the benefits it comes with. Upon knowing the wide array of advantages from fasting, I decided I will do it for physical, mental, and spiritual purposes. Together with my then 63-year-old mother and a friend, we embarked on a 5-day water-only fast with some apple cider vinegar for potassium and salt water for sodium. We went about our normal day with our usual tasks, and we succeeded with ease. We all lost a good amount of fats and the most dramatic would be my friend's reversal of *hypertriglyceridemia* (from more than 2,500 down to only 230 after a month). Over time, we engaged in intermittent fasting and occasionally extending our fast. I lost a total of about 22-25 pounds from my last heaviest weight and I felt really good.

Aside from being very comfortable with my own body now, I also get a lot of compliments that I look a lot younger, possibly with my skin. And most importantly, I never get the need for antihistamine and intranasal steroids. My allergies became things of the past and I can easily hug my dogs and put make-up on without experiencing any itch.

I shared what I learned with the people closest to my heart and I am so happy that they too have started on this journey. I have people who are closest to me and grew up with who used to be overweight but now have normal BMI. There is another that is from size 6 who dropped to size 0, and one with a lifetime of acne problems but with smoother skin after. From diabetes and hypertension to no medication needed. And from uncomfortable, to now being happy in their own form. Like them, I want you to be free too, free from food dependence, free from being tagged as the one, free from the stigma that you will never have the chance to have that body you so aim to have. If my story isn't enough, you can find a lot of testimonials from real people online. Look up *"Low-Carb Feasting and Fasting Community"* on Facebook and you will be amazed at the hundreds of thousands of success stories members are sharing to inspire others. I do hope you can try this process not just for weight but for overall health. You will know for sure that it is no fad since nobody else can have an ulterior motive with you being at your healthiest. The main beneficiary is just you, plainly and exclusively you.

If somebody told me before that I can achieve what I have achieved now, there's no way I would ever believe it. Note though that after more than 4 years in this lifestyle, I have changed my goal from weight loss to optimum health with moderate to high muscle mass. I have worked out, increased my proteins, continued low carb and fasting, and is no longer fixated with the scale. This is because I realized that as much as drastic weight loss is possible, it is not the ultimate goal that can make me sustainably happy. It is the health and freedom from illness with the stamina to work for my dreams for myself and my family. Being a woman who may be pregnant anytime and soon be breastfeeding if everything goes well, I no longer obsess over the numbers in the scale, so long that I remain with my daily IF and clean eating. I do not know when there will be a possible repeat or have the need to do those very long extended fasts again, but the discipline, confidence, and mental clarity I got are something that I will always be grateful for.

Three years after the COVID pandemic started, I have never been tested positive despite multiple testing and most of all, I have never been confined in bed disabled due to sickness ever since I started this way of life.

The BMI and weight that I have now is within a healthy range, and that's just an expected outcome when you start this LCF way of life as well. Finally, the way I look, the way I see myself in the mirror, is already the person that I always felt to be inside.

It may be faster or slower with you, but trust that in time, you will have it too.

In summary, this is what I did in chronological order:

- Five days of water-only fast, with minimal water, vinegar and salt (lost 10 pounds, note that this is largely water loss from an initial very high carb and inflammatory food intake).

- Two weeks of approximately 16:8 clean IF, no simple sugars (kept 6 pounds of the weight loss).

- Did 11 days of water-only fast (lost another 15 pounds).

- Two weeks of 16 to 24-hour clean fast (maintained the total ~20 pounds weight loss, already on goal of 19-20 BMI score but with low muscle mass).

- Seven days water-only fast - (lost another 5 pounds but gained back after a feast from a week-long vacation).

- Maintenance of 19 to 20 hours IF/ OMAD lifestyle, trying my best to stick to a low carb but with occasional high carb intake. Incorporation of 24-36 hour fast after a feast or whenever I have a high-carb intake.

- From a previously impaired fasting blood glucose level of 110-115 mg/dL, it is now down to 79 mg/dL and an HbA1c of 5.3% (Diabetes cut off is 6.5%).

- IF is now my way of life as I have reached my target weight. I do cyclical EF for other purposes (*autophagy, anti-aging, in need of focus like passing my specialty board exam and immune boosting effects whenever I have flu*). I still do not have a regular physical activity, but I also do not avoid long walks, stairs and far parking lots.

- Since the publication of the first edition in 2019, I have undergone multiple Dry Fasting and the longest fast I did was a 7-day DF, followed by 7 day clean fast, for a total of 14 days. I have kept the fat loss for 3 years and decided to work on increasing my muscle mass through exercise and resistance training for about 6 months. When I achieved my goal, I continued with my LCF way of life and only extended my fast for special reasons.

- The last planned indulgence I made was during my sister's wedding in 2020 where she was very excited for the cocktails she prepared. That was 3 years ago, and so far, I intend to keep it as a good memory to cherish.

Overall, I feel like my best version yet and there is nothing I wish for you than to be the best version of you too.

CHAPTER 18

Fasting Thoughts and Tips

"Whether you think you can or you think you can't, you are right."

- Henry Ford

First, believe. And read the *words* below, out loud if possible, and you can claim them as your own.

If others can do it, I can too.

All good food can wait.

A large group of people worldwide are into fasting, be it for religious, health or philosophical reasons.

This may not be important to you, but even celebrities swear by it including *Hugh Jackman, Beyonce, Jennifer Lopez, Nicole Kidman, Benedict Cumberbatch, Ben Affleck,* and many more.

Before eating out of your window, ask yourself, *is this a nutritional eating or just an emotional eating*?

Always remember what certain foods make you feel. (*Like for me, eating sugary foods reactivates my allergic rhinoconjunctivitis. It gives me itchy eyes as well as a bloated stomach and return of cravings, making fasting hours even more difficult.*)

Don't compare yourself with other's weight loss pace. Compare yourself with your previous self. Even if you are not losing as much, be glad that as of this moment, you are no longer gaining more weight.

As they say, just mind your own plate.

Fasting and eating healthy has a multitude of benefits that goes beyond weight loss.

This is not a quick fix diet; this is a lifestyle that is sustainable as a permanent way of life.

Once you have done an extended fast, missing a meal or two or even a day becomes no big deal.

Fasting makes eating pleasurable by a hundred-fold. A meal becomes not just a meal but a celebration of life. If you engage in OMAD, imagine a feeling of unique eating pleasure and celebration each day.

When fasting, you become much more focused and your attention to detail accelerates. I find it best to do my surgeries in a fasted state.

Eating sweet foods, even low carb sweeteners, can trigger sugar addiction for those affected. Thus, it is a big no-no during fasting and must be done with caution during your eating window.

Do not risk what you have achieved just because you felt emotional and needed food. Try drinking water first and go for a 10-minute walk with fresh air and see how it works.

Fasting allows you to do guilt-free feasting on momentous occasions with loved ones.

Only you have the power to give this gift to yourself.

Physical appearance is not everything that matters, but our own personal image about how we see ourselves does.

Let yourself be the representative of the real and ideal you.

Discipline is a state of mind.

Fasting is largely a mental exercise.

Practice your mental strength through fasting and by saying no to unhealthy foods.

The primary person who can benefit from all these is you.

Never stop believing, you can do it.

Give it at least two strict months before giving up totally.

What is two months as compared to a life-long benefit?

How do you feel about reversing signs of aging through fasting?

With proper guidance, how do you feel about the possibility of not needing maintenance medications anymore for allergies, asthma, diabetes, high cholesterol, and hypertension?

When you are fasting, you are in a protective and conservative mode. Your immune system is heightened, thus, protecting you from common illnesses like flu and cold.

I fast to heal my body.

I fast to improve my mind.

I fast for clarity and focus.

I fast for ideas.

I fast for healing, in all ways, pains and forms.

Fasting is being efficient, that includes no spending on extra food while I still have fats to burn.

The moment I eat, I become relaxed and instantly lose the critical thinking I had moments before I give in to food.

I can delay eating a certain food if my window is not yet open. But I can remember how it tastes simply because the foods that I like are the foods I have eaten many times before. The memory of its taste will be enough until my window opens.

And yes, you too can wait until your window opens.

Weight is only a small aspect of fasting. Do not be a slave of the weighing scale. Your body is likely reshaping and improving more than the scale can tell.

Try to move away from the scale until you finish the minimum two month cycle.

When fasting, your work productivity increases.

Do not be discouraged when the scale doesn't seem to move as much as you want it to. Trust the process because for some it takes time, and it is okay.

Have other gauge of improvement aside from scale, like a monthly mirror photo, how "honesty" pants/clothes fit, **how light you feel,** how radiant your skin has become and how others keep on commenting you are slimming down.

Do not mind others who are discouraging you from not eating. They may be concerned but they did not say a word when you were eating voraciously unhealthy foods 6 times a day before.

If others are giving negative comments about your practice and how you look "so skinny", try to assess first if there is genuine care from that person or just an uneducated opinion. Otherwise, if you see you are still in your healthy BMI range and are functioning well, you are good to go.

This is your own journey. If others will join, then well and good, but if there is no one else in your circle, keep on and remember that there is so much strength and reward in going and achieving solo.

Be patient.

A common reason for fasting failure is boredom and preoccupation with food. Be prepared and be productive. Plan your days ahead, best by doing something worthwhile or even by just binge- watching a very good TV series.

Join various support groups in social media, just type in keywords like Extended Fasting, intermittent fasting or one meal a day.

Download an app that tracks your daily fasting goals.

Reward yourself with non-food trophies after a successful fast or after achieving a certain goal.

Keep yourself busy during a planned fast.

Plan a productive activity during EF.

Strive for continued improvement and not perfection.

Be kind to yourself.

If all else fails, watch my YT videos at Dr. Josephine Grace Rojo Tan channel or send me a message and my team will be happy to help.

jgrtan@jgrtanmd.com   josephinegracechuarojo@gmail.com

CHAPTER 19

Other Benefits of Fasting

"I fast for greater physical and mental efficiency."

-Plato

It is said that weight loss is only a side effect of fasting, although a beneficial one at that. However, the real benefit of fasting occurs not in the visible scale but in a more significant and qualitative way. The following are the good effects of fasting in our health:

- Reduces risk of developing cancer and even shrinks certain tumors.

- Decreases allergic and inflammatory diseases such as allergic rhinitis, arthritis, joint pains, and even asthma.

- Unbelievable as it may seem, but when done right, fasting gives more energy and stamina to do heavier work.

- Reverses type II diabetes when done together with Low

Carb way of eating.

- Normalizes blood pressure for those with essential hypertension.
- Clears and heals skin diseases like acne eczema.
- Normalizes ovulation especially for women suffering from polycystic ovarian syndrome.
- Decreases bad cholesterol level and reduces arterial occlusion thereby decreasing risk for stroke and heart attack.
- Slows aging and promotes longevity through autophagy.
- Improves neurologic functioning.
- Decreases risk for developing neurodegenerative diseases such as Alzheimer's *disease*.

The details of each benefit and how to go about it is already beyond the scope of this book. It is included in the succeeding books of this series. Meantime, I believe that it is of great importance that we are all aware of such benefits. Now that you are knowledgeable with the basics of fasting and how it can improve our way of life, I encourage you to do your own readings and research so we can educate many more, especially those close to our hearts, and so we can get more out of this life TOGETHER.

CHAPTER 20

Summary and Pearls

"Fasting of the body is food for the soul."

-Saint John Chrysostom

Problem with weight management is not something that occurred overnight. One cannot just simply blame their own eating habits because it goes back more than that. In fact, it is only a manifestation of an underlying erroneous way of dealing with food that goes back for centuries already.

Like it or not, we are all a byproduct of upbringing by the multi-billion food industry that influenced our parents and grandparents to an eating pattern that is unnatural to humans. As our genetic make-up is still like that of our hunter-gatherer ancestors, we must embrace and incorporate fasting as our way of life. Without it, our body will keep on storing body fats until it can no longer accommodate it in its limited compartment and eventually disrupt our body's balance.

This disturbance in our metabolic homeostasis can then manifest as obesity, high blood pressure, diabetes, fatty liver, rapid aging, tumors and even death from stroke and heart attack. Thus, to start the healing process, we should strive to eliminate first the excess fat stores that we have and allow our body to refocus its energy, in order for it to repair itself. This is facilitated by fasting. Doing so will allow us to slowly burn the excess fats that we have been storing our whole life. Through extended fasting, one can safely achieve an ideal weight in the shortest possible time. I am pro-choice. Both IF and EF schedules can lead to **ketosis**, which is the fat-burning mode of our body and our aim in achieving our goal of an efficient weight loss process. In addition, we also identify clean fasting versus fat fasting, wherein, if you choose to engage in a clean fast, you are only allowed to consume water, black coffee, plain tea leaves, vinegar, and pure electrolytes like salt. Note that the only way to go with IF is through a clean fast for best results. However, when you decide to do an extended fast, you can have more liberty in your fluids should you decide to do EF through *fat fasting*. To recap, here's the difference between the following:

Extended fasting – Fasting for 24 hours or more. I advocate for everyone to try at least once in their life, engage in a 5 to 7-day EF when psychologically and physiologically ready. This will give you the most benefit in terms of weight loss, gastrointestinal system rest and a great mental boost for your future fasting schedules.

Clean Fasting – Drink sips of water only when feeling hungry or thirsty. You can have black coffee or plain tea. When feeling weak, take some salt by either taking it as is, or mix it in your drinks. I advise that you try to do clean fasting as long as you can. I did it for 11 days and stopped only when I already felt some cramps on my legs as I walked up a ramp. Too bad, I didn't have magnesium and potassium supplements that time to counter it. But should you plan to do it for more than 7 days, I suggest that you do it prepared. Kindly refer back to Chapter 5 for a full list of electrolytes that u can take while on a clean fast.

Fat Fasting – Previously termed as *dirty fasting*, reserve this in times when you can no longer sustain a clean fast. It is where you can consume calorie containing foods rich with healthy fats and nutrients that can help some sustain an EF. This would include vegetable and bone broth, MCT oil, pure coconut oil, butter, heavy creams, and whole full fat milk in limited amounts.

Intermittent fasting – This is when you fast for less than 24 hours. It may take some time before one is fully adjusted to IF. But I find that after about three days or so of headache, weakness and extreme cravings, people who are used to breakfast generally adapt well on the fourth day and those who are used to skipping breakfast adapts even better. A clean fast is encouraged during IF. You can slowly decrease your *"eating window"* from 12 hours to 4-5 hours or as desired. Remember that a bottle of beer or a glass of wine already constitutes "food" and should not be taken lightly.

Fasting, whether IF or EF is the core of managing weight and best if in conjunction with Low Carb. For optimum health, I suggest to maximize the benefits by eating the right foods when you can. The best foods to eat during a window period will depend on you. To be on the safe side, I believe in the science behind a Low Carbohydrate diet, wherein you avoid carbo-loaded foods that are not natural to the large part of human development, like breads, pasta, mashed potato, rice and noodles, especially when you haven't reached your goal weight yet. More important than those high carb whole foods, you must avoid processed foods full of preservatives and simple sugars as in table sugar, or those incorporated in items like in desserts, colas, fruit juices, blended coffees and other drinks. While you are still in the initial phase of trying to lose weight, it is best to avoid fruits as they are mostly full of fructose. Safe fruits would include avocado, coconut, and berries. For those who have sugar addiction or are always craving for sweets and chocolates, it is a good opportunity to practice avoidance and rehabilitate your palate away from the addicting taste. However, if this is not yet your time to do so, know that there are so many easy low-carb chocolate recipes online available for free. Just ask Google. ☺

As long as you are not pregnant, breastfeeding or a growing child, you can certainly fast! For those with medical conditions, kindly ask your trusted physician for advice first prior to engaging in such.

Once you have decided to proceed with fasting, you must also know when to break it. Although it is common to overeat after a fast, it is also noticeable that long-term faster knows the importance of breaking a fast slowly. And breaking the fast gently is really the way we should do it.

For special days, holidays, and vacations, you can certainly enjoy these precious moments both with food and family. Weight loss plateaus or even weight gain after a weight loss should not become a concern because you already know what to do and when to need to do it.

Trust the process and you will certainly attain the ideal healthy weight and optimum health you've always been dreaming of.

CHAPTER 21

Frequently Asked Questions

I believe that reading the book from cover to cover will give enlightenment to common questions. And sometimes, it is good to re-read either the whole book or certain chapters after you have already adapted to fasting as a way of life. However, for any gray area that this book may have, kindly send me a personal message and I welcome it with open arms. Whether it is a suggestion, a question, or a need for improvement, I consider it a pleasure and an opportunity to make this better.

This chapter will be updated from time to time. As of this writing, the following are the FAQs:

Is fasting the same as starving?
No, because fasting is a deliberate, conscious, and unforced decision of not consuming any calorie-containing foods for a specific period. The person who is fasting can choose to stop it at any time he/she wishes to. It is commonly done for health, religious, and philosophical reasons.

When will I know if I need to take electrolytes during an extended fast?
Each electrolyte abnormality will present differently. Weakness during the early days of fasting is commonly due to sodium depletion, thus, you can take in some salt little by little, not going more than 3 teaspoons per day. Whereas cramps may mean low in potassium and/or magnesium on the later days. See Chapter 5 for details.

How will I know when I will break my fast?
Kindly go back to Chapter 11 for the specifics. However, it is best to know your health status by checking your BMI and Body Fat Percentage does not go below normal while correlating it with how your body feels. Always listen to your body and do not risk anything life threatening just for the sake of weight loss. Remember that you can always fast again, should you feel the need to cut a planned EF.

Is extended fasting a requirement to lose weight?
Easy answer is no. Though, this depends on your goal and how would you like to go about it. If you are like me and my sister who wanted to test the waters right in, and see how we would perform, and see results significantly per day, then EF is for you. But for weight loss per se, it is not necessary. There are numerous success stories even just with 12 hours of daily IF alone and low carb, it can be done already.

After about 2 weeks in this lifestyle, I feel light but the scale doesn't seem to move nor I look slimmer, is this okay?

Yes, it is okay. Remember that it is important to give it at least two months before you can really see substantial and visible results. However, you may in fact feel lighter because you are losing fats that are not visibly obvious but are very important to your health. These are visceral fats or the dangerous fats that surround your internal organs like your liver, heart and intestines. Thus, do not worry and fast on!

I tried IF before and I cannot tolerate the headache and I am afraid I might faint. Can I really do it?

If you are not part of those identified in Chapter 7, I believe you certainly can. Acknowledge that the headache and light-headedness are common side-effects of the transition from the process of sugar/glucose-burning to fat-burning state. And can easily be corrected with the Salt Fix. You have the option to relax during these times for you to feel at ease, but you can also make yourself busy and preoccupied with something worthwhile to take your mind off it. Although there is in fact science behind these challenges, it also has a remedy (like electrolytes or rest). And it is not an exaggeration when we say that fasting is largely a challenge to mental strength rather than a physical one.

Why is it that my face looks slimmer but my stomach still looks bloated?

You may be fasting the right way, which is, getting into ketosis and fat-burning state. But it is time that you have to take a look at what you have been eating during your eating window. Remember, to achieve the maximum benefit, you have to pair fasting with the right healthy foods, especially whole, raw, unprocessed or the least processed foods. Sugary and carbohydrate-rich foods tend to hold more water than fats and proteins. Thus, this water retention may be the cause of your persistent abdominal weight and *bloating*.

Is it okay to overeat during my window?
Yes and no. Studies show that even if you feel like you overeat during your window, the amount you consume is still less than the amount you could have consumed if you have eaten 3 times a day on a regular breakfast- lunch-dinner routine. So, you can say it is "okay", although it is not advisable to really overeat during your window. It is again important to listen more to your body and just eat until you are satisfied. And even if in a way it is "not okay", it is expected during the first weeks of getting into this lifestyle, and you will just be surprised when time comes you suddenly get full even before you finish your planned feast. Overtime, I hope your feast will be trimmed down into a meal but still with a sense of satisfaction similar to that of a feast!

What is your recommended IF schedule?
It will depend on your goal. If you are still starting this way of life (WOL) and in the period of adjusting, I recommend you lengthen it as long as you can. From 12 hours, you can try to reach a minimum of 16-18 hours for you to have a substantial effect. Believe it or not, you will soon realize that a 6-8 hour window period is just a long time to allow us to eat. You will see that food is something that takes so much energy to process and a longer fasting period means more efficient time for your body to burn what you ate and tap the fat stores you are yet to burn. As

for maintenance, I personally believe in OMAD mixed with TMAD in a week, to not jeopardize our metabolism.

Is exercise necessary for weight loss?
As per Chapter 15, the answer is no. But exercise is best for other reasons like building muscles, endurance, and strength. The advantages are at maximum when done together with fasting and when you already achieved your target weight.

For females, how do you sustain fasting when you have your period?
Although female hormones are at the lowest during the menstrual period, none of it directly affects your metabolism and functioning. With adequate fluid and electrolyte intake and mental practice, fasting can be done safely and efficiently.

Can you continue working while fasting?
As I have mentioned many times, I am a doctor working in a very busy public hospital for 10-24 hours daily during the peak of my EFs. I perform surgeries for 4-12 hours straight while still fasting and nobody can tell the difference because I am functioning similarly or even better than when I was not fasting.

Once I achieve my target weight, can I stop fasting and go back to eating the "usual" way?
You can certainly do so but chances are, you will also go back to your previous body before you started it all. Thus, if you want a

lasting effect, you must acknowledge that this is not a one-time deal, but a lifestyle we as humans should embrace. Maintenance of IF that suits your schedule and occasional cyclical EF as part of one's routine saves time, money and resources and mealtime during an eating window.

Can I recommend this way of life to others?
Yes, you can definitely recommend this way of life to others, provided you know the basic do's and don'ts. However, know that no matter how good your intentions are, some people will react very negatively about it and will even humiliate you. Thus, a word of advice, choose wisely who you share this knowledge with and make sure you are confident enough to answer whatever questions they may throw. But to be safe, why not just recommend reading this book instead? I would really appreciate that. ☺

REFERENCES/SUGGESTED READINGS:

1. htttps://www.who.int/news-room/fact- sheets/detail/the-top-10-causes-of-death

2. https://siimland.com/everything-about- getting-enough-electrolytes-while-fasting/

3. http://siimland.com/keto-if-fasting/

4. Cahill Jr, G.F., 2006. Fuel metabolism in starvation. Annu. Rev. Nutr., 26, pp.1-22.

5. Castellini, M.A. and Rea, L.D., 1992. The biochemistry of natural fasting at its limits. Experientia, 48(6), pp.575-582.

6. Izumida, Y., Yahagi, N., Takeuchi, Y., Nishi, M., Shikama, A., Takarada, A., Masuda, Y., Kubota, M., Matsuzaka, T., Nakagawa, Y. and Iizuka, Y., 2013. Glycogen shortage during fasting triggers liver–brain–adipose neurocircuitry to facilitate fat utilization. Nature communications, 4, p.2316.

7. Sarah C. Couch (7 April 2006). "Ask an Expert: Fasting

and starvation mode". University of Cincinnati (NetWellness). Archived from the original on 19 July 2011

8. Anton, S.D., Moehl, K., Donahoo, W.T., Marosi, K., Lee, S.A., Mainous III, A.G., Leeuwenburgh, C. and Mattson, M.P., 2018. Flipping the metabolic switch: understanding and applying the health benefits of fasting. Obesity, 26(2), pp.254-268.

9. https://universityhealthnews.com/daily/ nutrition/leptin-foods-answer-always- hungry/

10. Stephens, Gin. Delay: Don´t Deny, Living an Intermittent Fasting Lifestyle

11. Fung, J. The Obesity Code: Unlocking the Secrets of Weight Loss

12. Fung J, Moore J. The Ultimate Guide to Fasting: Heal Your Body Through Intermittent, Alternate Day and Extended Fasting.

13. The Magic Pill at https://www.netflix.com/

14. https://www.medicalnewstoday.com/ articles/306638.ph

15. https://www.delish.com/food/g22617665/ celebrities-intermittent-fasting/

16. https://idmprogram.com/refeeding- syndromes-fasting-20/

17. https://www.allaboutfasting.com/breaking- a-fast.html

18. Mellanby, Kenneth (July 1942). "Metabolic Water and Desiccation". Nature. 150 (3792): 21. Bibcode:1942Natur.150...21M. doi:10.1038/150021a0. S2CID 4089414.

19. ^ Morrison, S. D. (1953-11-28). "A method for the calculation of metabolic water". The Journal of Physiology. 122 (2): 399–402. doi:10.1113/jphysiol.1953.sp005009. ISSN 0022-3751. PMC 1366125. PMID 13118549.

20. ^ Medicine, Institute of; Board, Food Nutrition; Intakes, Standing Committee on the Scientific Evaluation of Dietary Reference; Water, Panel on Dietary Reference Intakes for Electrolytes and (2005). 4 Water | Dietary Reference Intakes for Water, Potassium, Sodium, Chloride, and Sulfate | The National Academies Press. p. 85. doi:10.17226/10925. ISBN 978-0-309-09169-5.

21. "Racing the wind. Water economy and energy expenditure in avian endurance flight". Archived from the

original on 2008-06-29. Retrieved 2008-08-01.

22. ^ Klaassen M (1996). "Metabolic constraints on long-distance migration in birds". J Exp Biol. 199 (Pt 1): 57–64. doi:10.1242/jeb.199.1.57. PMID 9317335.

23. ^ Jump up to:a b Board on Agriculture and Natural Resources (BANR), Nutrient Requirements of Nonhuman Primates: Second Revised Edition (2003), p. 144. [1]

APPENDIX A

Different 20-gram carbohydrates

Different perspectives on how a **20-gram carbohydrates** *will look like*

https://www.dietdoctor.com/low-carb/20-50- how-much

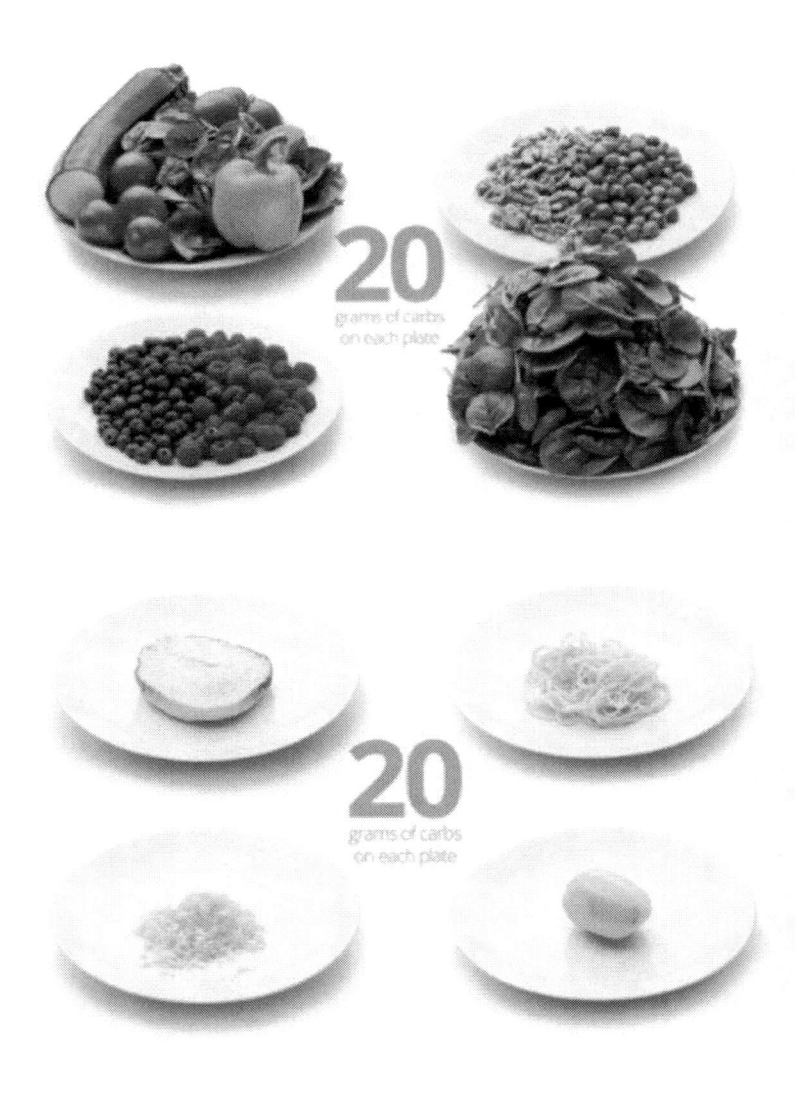

APPENDIX B

Basal Metabolic Index Chart

WEIGHT lbs	100	105	110	115	120	125	130	135	140	145	150	155	160	165	170	175	180	185	190	195	200	205	210	215
kgs	45.5	47.7	50.0	52.3	54.5	56.8	59.1	61.4	63.6	65.9	68.2	70.5	72.7	75.0	77.3	79.5	81.8	84.1	86.4	88.6	90.9	93.2	95.5	97.7
HEIGHT in/cm	Underweight					Healthy					Overweight					Obese					Extremely obese			
5'0" · 152.4	19	20	21	22	23	24	25	26	27	28	29	30	31	32	33	34	35	36	37	38	39	40	41	42
5'1" · 154.9	18	19	20	21	22	23	24	25	26	27	28	29	30	31	32	33	34	35	36	37	38	39	39	40
5'2" · 157.4	18	19	20	21	22	22	23	24	25	26	27	28	29	30	31	32	33	34	35	36	37	37	38	39
5'3" · 160.0	17	18	19	20	21	22	23	24	25	26	26	27	28	29	30	31	32	33	34	35	36	36	37	38
5'4" · 162.5	17	18	19	20	21	21	22	23	24	25	26	27	28	28	29	30	31	32	33	34	35	35	36	37
5'5" · 165.1	16	17	18	19	20	21	22	22	23	24	25	26	27	28	28	29	30	31	32	33	34	34	35	36
5'6" · 167.6	16	17	18	19	19	20	21	22	23	24	24	25	26	27	28	28	29	30	31	32	33	33	34	35
5'7" · 170.1	15	16	17	18	19	20	20	21	22	23	24	24	25	26	27	27	28	29	30	31	31	32	33	34
5'8" · 172.7	15	16	17	18	18	19	20	21	22	22	23	24	25	25	26	27	28	28	29	30	30	31	32	33
5'9" · 175.2	14	15	16	17	18	19	19	20	21	21	22	23	24	24	25	26	27	27	28	29	30	30	31	32
5'10" · 177.8	14	15	16	17	17	18	19	19	20	21	22	22	23	24	25	25	26	27	27	28	29	29	30	31
5'11" · 180.3	14	15	15	16	17	18	18	19	20	20	21	22	22	23	24	25	25	26	27	27	28	29	29	30
6'0" · 182.8	13	14	15	16	16	17	18	18	19	20	20	21	22	22	23	24	24	25	26	26	27	28	28	29
6'1" · 185.4	13	14	14	15	16	16	17	18	18	19	20	20	21	22	22	23	24	24	25	26	26	27	28	28
6'2" · 187.9	12	13	14	14	15	16	17	17	18	19	19	20	21	21	22	23	23	24	25	25	26	26	27	28
6'3" · 190.5	12	13	13	14	15	15	16	17	18	18	19	19	20	21	21	22	23	23	24	24	25	26	26	27
6'4" · 193.0	12	12	13	14	14	15	16	16	17	17	18	19	20	20	21	21	22	23	23	24	25	25	26	26

APPENDIX C

Sample Intermittent Fasting Schedules

First Meal	Last Meal	Eating Window	Total Fasting
9AM	5PM	8 Hours	16 Hours
10AM	6PM	8 Hours	16 Hours
11AM	7PM	8 Hours	16 Hours
12NN	7PM	8 Hours	16 Hours
12NN	6PM	7 Hours	17 Hours
12NN	5PM	6 Hours	18 Hours
1PM	6PM	5 Hours	19 Hours
1PM	5PM	4 Hours	20 Hours
2PM	6PM	4 Hours	20 Hours
3PM	7PM	4 Hours	20 Hours
3PM	8PM	5 Hours	19 Hours
4PM	9PM	5 Hours	19 Hours

APPENDIX D

Sample Short-term EF Schedules

Type	TIME	8AM	12NN	4PM	6PM	8PM
42H Fast 3x per week	Day 1	Fast	Eat	Eat	Eat	Fast
	Day 2	Fast	Fast	Fast	Fast	Fast
	Day 3	Fast	Eat	Eat	Eat	Fast
	Day 4	Fast	Fast	Fast	Fast	Fast
	Day 5	Fast	Eat	Eat	Eat	Fast
	Day 6	Fast	Fast	Fast	Fast	Fast
	Day 7	Fast	Eat	Eat	Eat	Fast

Type	TIME	8AM	12NN	4PM	6PM	8PM
ADF or 36hr Fast	Day 1	Fast	Fast	Fast	Fast	Fast
	Day 2	Eat	Eat	Eat	Eat	Eat
	Day 3	Fast	Fast	Fast	Fast	Fast
	Day 4	Eat	Eat	Eat	Eat	Eat
	Day 5	Fast	Fast	Fast	Fast	Fast
	Day 6	Eat	Eat	Eat	Eat	Eat
	Day 7	Fast	Fast	Fast	Fast	Fast

APPENDIX E

#JGCRojoFoodList

Josephine Grace Rojo Tan, MD

Facial Plastic & Rhinoplasty Surgery
Diseases of the Ears, Nose and Throat – Head & Neck Surgery Root
Cause Medicine | Low Carb Nutrition and Fasting Lifestyle

Manila | Cebu | Bacolod
Clinic Hours: By Appointment

+63 917 993 12 39
Follow: FB | YouTube | IG | T

Safe

Can be eaten as much as you can so long as you do not pair it with the ones in Caution and Danger list. A mixture of both fats and proteins can be eaten together. Avoid eating pure proteins only.

Meats & Poultry Products – Pork, Beef, Chicken, Lamb, Turkey, Duck, Eggs, Carabao, Goat/Mutton, Rabbit Meat, Horse, Kangaroo, other animal meats, liver & organs.

Vegetables – All green leafy vegetables, Eggplant, Cucumber, Peppers, Asparagus, Cauliflower, Broccoli, Cabbage, Pechay, Lettuce, Malunggay, Spinach, Kangkong, Spring Onions, Radishes, Mushrooms

Oil & Fats – Coconut Oil, Olive Oil, Avocado Oil, Ghee, Lard, Tallow, Fish Oil, Grass-fed butter, MCT (Limit Omega 6)

Seafood – fish (choose high in Omega 3, less mercury), crustaceans, shells, seaweeds, oysters, shrimp, crabs, eel

Low Carb Fruits – seasonal Avocado, Berries, Mature Coconut Meat, Tomato, Olives, Lemon, Calamansi

Nuts and Seeds – Almonds, Pecan, Walnut, Macadamia, Brazil, Pine Nuts, Sunflower Seeds, Pumpkin seeds and other seeds (2-3x a week)

Spices – Cinnamon, B&W Peppers, Paprika, Nutmeg, Chili Powders and others are okay provided they do not contain sugar or processed oils.

Salt – Himalayan pink salt, natural sea/table salt, rock salt

Natural Vinegar – coconut, sugar cane, Apple Cider, Red Wine, Rice Vinegar, etc.

Flour Alternative: Almond, Coconut Flour, Oat Fiber, Wheat Vital Gluten Other Baking needs: Psyllium Husk Powder, Xanthan Gum, Flaxseed Powder, Chia Seeds, Shirataki/Konjac derivatives

Other drinks: (ALL Plain/Unsweetened) coffee, tea or cocoa, Water with lemon zest, cucumber, herbs, mint or peppermint leaves, almond milk

Others: Sesame Seeds, Baking Soda, Xanthan Gum, Psyllium Husk, Baking Powder, Cream of Tartar (as needed, with indication)

Caution

Take with caution, limit to only 1 serving a day. Carbo intake should be limited to 20-50g/day. Zero calorie sw can trigger sugar addiction. Alcoholic drinks can lead to Processed meats, hydrogenated oils, and soy product inflammatory when taken in excess.

With Insulin Effect:

Fruits – MAJORITY of fruits (i.e. apples, mango & b

Crops & Starchy Foods – Carrots, Potato, Sweet Pot Taro, Ube, Squash, Pumpkin, Peanuts, Beans

Grains - Oats, Wheat, Corn, Rice, Quinoa (limit to 2

With Unnatural Cravings/Inflammatory Effect:

Processed Meats – Bacon, Chorizo, Ham, Salami, P Tocino, Canned Fish & Meat products

Processed Cheese & Dairies – Regular Butter, most soft & hard cheeses, heavy cream

Condiments & Flavorings – Coco aminos, Mayo, Ket Sauces, Dips, Vanilla Syrup, Fruit flavors

Zero Calorie, Zero Carb Sweeteners & Drinks – Allul Stevia, Monkfruit, Erythritol, Zero Colas, arti keto/low-carb desserts, Aspartame, Sucralose, etc

Soy Products – Soy Sauce, Tofu, Soy Milk

Stalls weight-loss/fat-burning/Toxic to Liver:

Alcoholic drinks – Wine, Vodka, Rum, Whiskey
Others: All Purpose Cream including Vegan Cream

Danger

Must be avoided as much as you can.

Ultra-Processed Foods - Pastries, pasta, chips, de Cakes, Ice creams, Candies, Breads, Baked pro French fries, corn/potato chips, sugared meat

Sugar – brown, coco sugar, agave, honey, corn syr

Processed Oils & Condiments – Canola, sunflowe hydrogenated vegetable oils, margarine, shorte

Worst Drinks – sodas, fruit juices, beer, milk tea &

APPENDIX F

Let's Start This Journey Together

Start by writing down your goals like desired weight, BMI, waist/hips/arm measurements or body fat percentage, or even some "non-scale victory" (NSV) like fitting back to a smaller dress. Trust that you can achieve it. After knowing all the details on fasting and low-carbohydrate diet, you are now ready to design your own routine. If not, let me give you two ways to do it.

The first approach is the fast, jumpstart approach wherein you directly indulge into a minimum of five days fasting to ensure that you will be in full ketosis by the time you break your fast. This is how we started in our family. As we are convinced that we can do it, we have each other to support one another. We also choose to have this in a normal week with no extra physically draining tasks. At work, I have informed my workmates that I am on an extended fast and even asked my superior that I will be converting my lunch- break to a resting break should I ever feel lightheaded or in need to rest. Surprisingly, that did not come. Except for mouth dryness and occasional weakness, we feel as normal as we can be. The weakness was instantly relieved by intake of water with salt and some apple cider vinegar for potassium and sodium. The hunger that happens 2-3x a day persisted, but the intensity keeps getting smaller and smaller each day. Whenever there's food temptations, instead of avoiding them, I savor their smell and I convince myself that I know how they taste so well because I've tasted them many times before and I can eat it any time after, but right at that moment, I am in the most crucial time of making something better out of myself. I am in the process of becoming my best version. I think to myself, *"What is one week as compared to a lifetime that I have spent indulging in food with regrets after which led me to a body type I so wanted to improve?"*, *"Or the optimum health and physique that I can achieve from this point onwards?"*. You may have doubts but remember, there is no shame in trying. The fact that you are open to making good changes with your life, starting with your commitment to better health, is already commendable.

If at any point you feel tired, you can rest at any time, or stop at any time and start again when you are ready. There was even a time where I had planned for a week-long fast but ended up doing a 24 or 40 hour fast instead simply because I listened to my body. There is no need to rush if you feel you are already unsure of yourself. However, should you feel positive about it, you can do the following:

Day 1 to 3- Clean, water-only fasting, may have salt and approved fluids.

Days 3 to 6 - Continue clean fasting, may take a multivitamin with electrolytes if deemed necessary. If it is not enough, you can proceed with *fat fasting* like having a bulletproof coffee, bone broth, and others as previously specified.

Day 7 - If you can no longer extend it beyond seven days, slowly break your fast by eating vegetable soup first, and after an hour, a light meal before you eat a proper low carbohydrate meal. Limit your eating window to only 5 hours when you can. Eat mindfully and pleasurably. However, if you feel you can still go another day, you can freely do so.

- Day 8 onwards - You can do 16 or 18 hours daily intermittent fasting for weeks doing strictly a low carb diet.

- Day 21 - You may repeat another cycle of extended fast or continue IF or engage on OMAD until you reach your desired goal. Mix it with TMAD 2-3x in a week to avoid adaptation. Just trust the process, because slowly yet surely, you will get there even with or without exercise.

The second approach is mostly followed by my friends whom I don't see on a day-to-day basis, to which the daily encouragement and monitoring is somewhat limited, as compared to my family who I live with. If you have never heard of IF and are doubtful on how this is going to work out, you can start by slowly extending your overnight fast. As explained earlier, make it into a goal to have at least 12 hours of fasting daily. You can have one light meal to open your window, have a proper meal in between, and another light meal to close it. Or you can have two proper meals upon opening and another one before closing your "*eating window*", with nothing but coffee, tea, or water in between the two meals. Follow this routine for at least two months and see the difference yourself. Some may not have significant weight loss per se, but people will start to notice how your face and body slowly improves in shape, including clearer skin, more toned structure, and lighter appearance. Common non-scale benefits include decreased inflammation, joint pains, and even allergies. The moment you graduate from a month of IF, you can level up to OMAD and even try extended fasting slowly in time.

I know it is much easier if you have a support group as you decide to embark on this journey, but you must accept the fact that there is a possibility that you might be going through this alone, and you must persist despite the circumstances. You will be the one who will reap the benefits after all. Right now, we have a support (closed) group on Facebook where you are most welcome to join. Just look for the group named **Low-Carb Feasting and Fasting Community** and **Life Without Rice**. You can also join various international support groups online where people openly support each other's journey.

Always be psychologically prepared that sometimes, the people closest to you will be the ones discouraging or tempting you to break your fast or eat the sugary snacks while you are doing your best to resist. Know your goals and know yourself. Make these two months a test of self-love and a beginning of self-care your body has been craving for.

In the beginning, I found it beneficial that I cleaned out my pantry first. I gave away all the simple sugars, biscuits, and juices that I have. Then, I bought a week's supply of cabbage and eggs as my staple. I downloaded the app LIFE for fasting to keep track of my daily fast during the first 3 years. I placed the food list on the dining table. I made a daily routine for going to work early and getting myself busy during the day. As a result, I sleep regularly earlier than I used to. During the weekends or during idle times when I cannot help but think about food, I fill up my time watching binge-worthy shows or some *YouTube* videos on the benefits of fasting and related videos like "how to fast successfully". Aside from enriching my knowledge, it successfully helped me to overcome one cycle of almost 11 days, one cycle of seven days and many more cycles of fasting.

I was a sugar and food addict. *Coke* has been like water. And I was raised in an environment where the definition of fullness is when you can no longer breathe deeply or sit straight. I used to eat very quickly and the only parts I love eating in cakes are the frosting. But now, I am far from where I used to be. And I feel like I already got my share of carb indulgence one is expected to have in a lifetime that I no longer crave eating it even if it is in front of me. But to be honest, I know that is impossible. I no longer give in to sugars and just fast right after. If a craving for sweets appears, I do the following remedies: The Salt Fix with vinegar or eat low carb desserts. If you choose to take real sugar, you can have sweets with the frequency like that of a seasoned fruit or the chance of finding honey in the wild. But realistically speaking, sweets are already part of our modern day and varieties of fruits are practically available all year round. You can have it, but timing and amount is the key. Something that I do not want to play around with, that is why it is full abstinence for me. So long as you strike a balance between regular eating patterns, occasional feast, and planned fast, you can achieve the health and physique our hunter-gatherer ancestors used to have.

I will leave the decision to you on how you will go about it. You can start strong with extended fast and maintain on OMAD to TMAD - what I consider to be the most effective and the most efficient. Or you can slowly ease in with increasing IF and OMAD while eating whatever you can, especially incorporating sugars during your window with caution. Again, there is no such thing as perfection that is uniform for everyone, but there is always something that is perfect for you, and time is in your hands for you to learn it little by little each day. Feel free to experiment and see for yourself what works for you and the life you plan to have.

Again, add me on Facebook, follow me on Instagram, subscribe to my YouTube channel or send me an email and I'd be more than willing to help as soon as time allows.

APPENDIX G

List and Recipe of Easy, Affordable

Low Carb, High Fiber Alternatives

Buttered Bland Greens - Use finely chopped cabbage, broccoli and/or cauliflower and sauté it in butter. You can mix it with whatever food you fancy on the above green list. The more common they are, the better your compliance will be. The longer you cook them, the lesser they taste, thus the more palatable they become. However, if you are used to their raw taste, you can eat them just as soon as the butter melts to maximize intake of the nutrients.

High Fiber Omelets - You can use whole eggs or just the white and cook the yolk separately and serve as a different side dish. For a single full serving, you can beat 1-2 eggs and add 2-4 cups of chopped greens and that's it, to be paired with your main fatty meat. An alternative would be two tablespoons of ground flaxseed meal or *psyllium* husk powder. You can add cheese, cream cheese, coconut flour or almond flour, whatever is available and depending on your preferred consistency. This is very filling and a perfect match to any meat.

Fresh salads - Lettuce, finely chopped cabbage and bell peppers, cucumber, tomato, all mixed together or alone, with homemade mayo, some salt, and a teaspoon of vinegar is just one of our table staples. These are very easy to buy and to prepare without the need for cooking! Olive oil is the best oil to use for salads.

Noodles and Pasta without the Carbs - Whether it's a chicken or beef soup, or red or white pasta dish, just cook it as is but replace the noodles and pasta with steamed cauliflower or fine strips of vegetables. With these, you won't be missing any of them anymore. Cook in pure coconut cooking oil or butter or lard.

These are just samples and my favorite ones because they are very cheap, don't spoil easily, delicious, and very easy to prepare. Fiber is optional; proteins and fats especially coming from meat are not. You can explore by adding in other low-carb items you like and create your own.

APPENDIX H

Low Carbohydrate Dessert

There are thousands of easy low carb desserts available online, but two of my favorites are as follows:

Dark Chocolate - Just mix 1 cup of 100% pure cocoa, 250 grams of cream cheese, and five tablespoons of Monk fruit sweetener and pour into chocolate bar molds or even small cupcake cups. If you add one cup of heavy cream, it will be converted into a chocolate pudding. Chill and serve.

Avocado Ice Cream - Puree four cups of sliced avocado, add 250gms heavy cream and four tablespoons Monk fruit sweetener or stevia counterpart. Chill and serve.

There are hundreds more, but to cure a sweet tooth and silence the chocolate monster within, a bite of these treats surely fits.

APPENDIX I

Low Carb Cooking and Baking

For those who are fond of baking, there are a lot of common ketogenic counterparts on the internet. Once you've mastered the art of having low carbohydrate dishes, you can maximize the benefit by converting it into a healthy low carb meal, where those alternatives are paired with a healthy fatty main course. Examples would include pork, salmon, lamb, and many more. Refer to the green list for the foods you can eat and the red list as the items you should avoid. Although calorie counting is not really recommended, but by proportion, 50-70% of your energy foods can come from fats, 30-45% from proteins, and 5% from carbs. That 5% of carbs are usually less than 20 to 50 grams per day. Start reading labels if you buy processed foods and avoid those with carbohydrate or sugar content more than one gram per serving or greater than 5-10 grams per 100 grams, unless it's the only thing you will consume for the day.

APPENDIX J

DCR Protocol

DCR Protocol is a fasting protocol that Dr. Grace personally designed, with the aim of healing like that of the challenging Phoenix Protocol, while considering the average working schedule of adults, mental ease and most importantly, safety.

DCR stands for Dry, Clean and Refeeding. This is a cycle of one day Dry Fasting, followed by second day of Clean Fasting and third day of high-protein refeeding. This is repeated for at least 7 times, amounting to 21 days if done continuously, or 24 days if done twice in a week. Note that DCR is recommended only for experienced fasters, especially those who have tried at least one 48 hours of clean fasting and 24 hours of dry fasting to appreciate this process.

For those who are mentally ready, the following DCR Protocol is recommended by the author:

- Sunday 6:00 PM:
    - Last water and food intake
- Monday:

- Cycle 1 Dry Fasting (DF)
- No water and any other oral intake.
- One can take a bath and brush teeth but not swallow anything.
- May do exercise in the morning as tolerated.
- Best to be mentally busy during this time but avoid exposure to humid environments and excessive sweating to avoid dehydration.
- If one cannot be productive, then a rest and sleep may also be done.
- Water, other fluids, and electrolytes may be taken as needed starting 6:00 PM to end the 24-hour DF. Take in sips and not in gulps.
- This day may be the hardest but the mental strength is still high since it is just the first day.
- Supplements like melatonin may be taken before bedtime.

- Tuesday:
  - Cycle 1 Clean Fasting (CF)
  - Water, plain coffee, tea using fresh or dried herbs, with salt and potassium may be taken.
  - After a day of DF, one can savor and appreciate water so much more.
  - Exercise is still optional but may be done with an

ample amount of electrolytes after sweating. Do it in the morning.

- Can be physically and mentally active during this day.
- Aim to break your fast at 6:00 PM to complete the 48 hours of fasting. But if not yet tolerated, be kind to yourself and break it earlier as needed.
- Have a light dinner with plain proteins and plan a relaxing night after.
- Sample breakfast at 6:00 PM would be a bone broth or simple soup, followed by eggs, chicken or white fish about 30 minutes after.
- Close your eating window about 4-6 hours before your intended bedtime and last water intake at two hours before sleeping.
- For those who are taking melatonin, take it 30 minutes before going to bed with sips of water.

- Wednesday
    - Cycle 1 Protein Refeeding (PF)
    - A 12-hour eating window may be maximized to properly nourish your body from the last two days of fasting and prepare it for the upcoming cycles of fasting.
    - High quality proteins with healthy fats are recommended, including grass-fed beef, organic pork, chicken, fish, shrimp and other seafood.

- o Vegetables are optional and should be taken last in a meal if included.
- o Avoid any form of starchy carbohydrates and simple sugars including low carb desserts.
- o This is a time to enjoy either alone or with loved ones.
- o Close your eating window by 6:00 PM. You may opt to delay it but know that you may have to delay your next day's water intake too.

- Thursday
  - o Cycle 2 Dry Fasting
  - o This day is similar to Monday.

- Friday
  - o Cycle 2 Clean Fasting
  - o This day is similar to Tuesday.
  - o Since Friday is usually a time when people go out, one may enjoy a night out with family and friends. Just make sure to stick to light proteins and sugar and alcohol-free drinks.

- Saturday and Sunday
  - o Cycle 2 Protein Refeeding
  - o This is similar to Wednesday but can be done in two days.
  - o This way, weekend gatherings can still resume and if

you do not wish to inform others, nobody can notice.

- End your feasting window by 6PM and repeat the following week for two and a half more weeks to complete a total of seven 7 cycles of DCR protocol.

The following parameters and laboratory examinations may be taken before the DCR protocol, a day after, two weeks after, and a month after to see the improvements:

1. Weight & BMI
2. Body Composition
3. Labs:
   a. CBC
   b. Urinalysis
   c. Lipid Profile
   d. SGPT
   e. SGOT
   f. Uric Acid
   g. Fasting Blood Sugar
   h. HbA1c – start and after 3 months
   i. ESR
   j. CRP

k. Electrolytes: Sodium and Potassium

  l. ECG – if with cardiac symptoms only

  m. Chest X-ray - optional

DCR Protocol has helped the author and many of her family and loved one's health with *leaky gut syndrome*, allergies, food intolerance, elevated cholesterol, elevated liver enzymes, and inflammation.

This protocol is not required but a good tool to know, should there come a time when one feels he needs it.

Author's Notes

To you,

By now, I hope you are done reading the whole book. I know there may still be doubts within you, especially with the uncertainty whether you can do it or not. I understand it is a lot to take in. But if there is a minimum take home message that I want everyone to have, it's these:

Fasting is a natural process.

It is okay not to eat all the time.

Unintentional skipped meals should not be a cause of worry but to be celebrated.

If EF is too much or unnecessary for you, then doing IF for as long as you can is the next best step.

Ketogenic diet, to some extent, biochemically mimics the effect of fasting through ketosis at a slower pace.

Can't let go of carbs? Compensate by fasting.

Can't afford an extended fast? Compensate by eating Low Carb meals.

Want to have the best results the fastest way? Do both!

When asked why you fast, just answer "It's because I can", with confidence.

Lastly, if you are asked by anybody what you are doing, in a limited time and avenue to explain things completely, then I humbly suggest for you to avoid talking about "fasting". Because they will probably just raise an eyebrow and close their minds even before you say another word. Instead, you can show them the results and wait until they are truly interested and have a proper time and place to talk about it substantially and completely. It is the main reason why fasting is not mentioned in the cover of the book, in hope that in the end, even a close-minded reader will have the acceptance that it is a natural part of human existence, whether or not he/she chooses to practice such.

If you think somebody else you care about can benefit from this book, pay it forward by sharing it with them or giving one as a gift. It will be my pleasure to help more.

Yours truly,

Grace

Made in the USA
Columbia, SC
09 February 2024